AF393628

Venous Disorders of the Legs

Springer

*London
Berlin
Heidelberg
New York
Barcelona
Budapest
Hong Kong
Milan
Paris
Santa Clara
Singapore
Tokyo*

L. L. Tretbar

Venous Disorders of the Legs

Principles and Practice

With 93 Figures
including 16 Color Plates

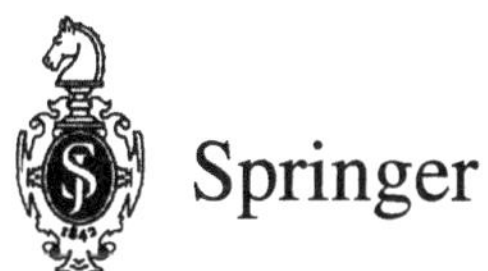

Springer

Lawrence L. Tretbar, MD, Professor, Clinical Surgery, University of Missouri – Kansas City School of Medicine
Phlebologic Institute of the Midwest, 8787 Ballentine, Shawnee Mission, Kansas 66214, USA

Cover illustrations: The insets show: Figure 7.3 (the Müller hook, the Oesch, the Ramelet, and the Tretbar hook); Figure 1.4 (the deep venous plexus of the foot outlined with dye).

British Library Cataloguing in Publication Data
Tretbar, Lawrence L.
 Venous disorders of the legs : principles and practice
 1. Veins – Diseases   2. Veins – Diseases – Treatment   3. Leg – Blood-vessels – Diseases
 I. Title
 616.1'4

Library of Congress Cataloging-in-Publication Data
Tretbar, Lawrence L., 1933–
 Venous disorders of the legs : principles and practice / L. L. Tretbar
  p. cm.
 Includes bibliographical references and index.

 ISBN-13: 978-1-4471-1203-7   e-ISBN-13: 978-1-4471-0795-8
 DOI: 10.1007/978-1-4471-0795-8

 1. Leg – Blood-Vessels – Diseases. 2. Varicose Veins. I. Title. [DNLM: 1. Varicose Veins.
 2. Leg – blood supply. 3. Venous Insufficiency. 4. Veins – physiopathology. WG 620 T799v 1998]
RC695.T74 1998
616.1'4 – dc21
DNLM/DLC   98–6341
for Library of Congress   CIP

Typeset by The Midlands Book Typesetting Company, Loughborough

28/3830-543210   Printed on acid-free paper

Foreword

Within the last five years a number of new books on venous disorders have been produced. Previously the study of venous disease was well-served by the classic texts of Foote, Anning, Dodd and Cockett, and Hobbs, but these texts are now out of print and out of date. How does Larry Tretbar's book equate with its competition? Those of you who pick up or purchase this delightful little book will not be disappointed. It is a single author text which is clearly written and succinct. In just over 100 pages Tretbar distils the work of many of his larger competitors without losing any vital information along the way. He also provides new insights and ideas in many areas. Contents are set out in a standard format but the writing is pithy and the line drawings (mostly by the author himself) are clear and helpful. It excels in the management and treatment of varicose veins where the author has made his major contribution. The book contains many of the classic venous references though these of necessity cannot be comprehensive in the interest of brevity.

Linton pointed out that diseases of the veins of the lower extremities are one of the commonest of human ailments that can be remedied by surgical measures. These disorders are often poorly managed by junior doctors who fail to acquaint themselves with the anatomy and pathophysiology of these disorders. For this reason I have no doubt that this monograph will find its way to the bookshelves of all those who are interested in the treatment of venous diseases, and I can specially recommend it to those who are starting to treat patients for the first time as it provides a comprehensive but readable guide to all that they need to know.

Professor K.G. Burnand
Professor of Vascular Surgery
St Thomas' Hospital
London

Preface

The preface to a book presents a wonderful opportunity for the author to let his hair down, to speak in ordinary English, to tell the story of his literary achievement and to let his supporters know just how much he appreciates them.

Although I have lectured and written journal articles on the topic of venous disease for many years, this book is the feature-length publication. It has allowed me to combine more than 30 years' of personal experience with that of others to create a primer with some depth and, I hope, a balanced view of this unique medical specialty.

My first real contact with the vascular system came during a year in my general surgery residency in which I worked as a Research Fellow for Dr Willem Kolff in his Department of Artificial Organs. Among the many medical devices Dr Kolff invented, the most famous is the artificial kidney which permits renal dialysis. With another young surgeon my year-long project was to design, build and implant an artificial heart into the chest of a calf. Here I quickly learned that the venous system was just as important to the organism as were its arteries. I learned about *vis a tergo*, *vis a fonte*, venous hypertension and the problems of venous return. Dr Kolff challenged us to create new approaches or concepts to solve a problem . . . and to make them work. It was a year of profound vascular experience.

My mentor during those years of residency was Dr George "Barney" Crile, the son of one of the founders of the Cleveland Clinic. Not only did he introduce modified radical mastectomy into American surgery but he inspired us to "question the time-honored ideas". He believed that any medical viewpoint more than five years old needed thorough re-evaluation. This concept has helped me place a new perspective on the traditional American attitudes toward varicose vein treatment.

My first contact with sclerotherapy was at the West Middlesex University Hospital in London during a year spent there as a Senior Registrar. The hospital's vein clinic, which I had to manage, was performing the Fegan technique of injection/compression for large varicose veins. I learned the technique and brought it back to the US, where it received little interest. Thirty years later almost every American doctor seems to be interested in sclerotherapy.

Mr George Fegan, the remaining "godfather" of contemporary phlebology, is still challenging us to consider the role of incompetent perforators in the treatment of varicose veins. I treasure his friendship and support.

Thanks are also due to Kathy, Kirsten and Eric who have spent many hours listening to tedious talk about veins and waiting for me to revise and edit; to my office staff, Marsha Stillions, Christa Stillions, Amy Hellige and my associate Dr Marcus Stanbro, who have adjusted their schedules to give me more time at the word processor. I appreciate Dr Ricardo Majia's diplomatic proof reading. Of course the staff at Springer-Verlag London have done their best to keep me in line and on time. Thanks Nick and Nick, Chris, Deirdre and Robin for your help.

L.L. Tretbar

Contents

CHAPTER 1

Anatomy of the Leg Veins

The structure and function of the venous system have been of special interest to anatomists for centuries. The veins are easily seen when diseased, especially those of the superficial system, and easily accessible to the anatomist. Nevertheless the true nature of the venous system remained a mystery for hundreds of years.

Galen in the 2nd century AD had clear insights into venous diseases and described treatments for venous ulcers and varicose veins. Unfortunately his erroneous views of the nature and function of blood pervaded scientific thought for 15 centuries. Galenic physiology held that blood was created in the liver where it received "natural spirits". It then was attracted, as if by centrifugal force, to the periphery of the body. Although it now seems simple to understand the function of the veins and their valves, it remained until the 17th century for the true nature of the venous system to be revealed.

With vivid and sometimes colorful imagination Vesalius, Fallopius and Leonardo da Vinci described the venous system. But it was Hieronymus Fabricius of Aquapendente, a student of Fallopius and himself a teacher of anatomy at the University of Padua, who gave the first accurate description of the venous valves. He knew that the valves helped regulate the flow of blood in veins but still held to Galen's mistaken notion of circulation. Nevertheless Fabricius' description of the valvular arrangement helped Harvey develop and support his own theory of circulation.

William Harvey, an English physician studying in Padua with Fabricius, finally explained the circulation of blood in 1628. In his famous explication, *Exercitatio anatomica de mortu cordis et sanguinis in animalibus* (Anatomic Treatise on the Motion of the Heart and Blood in Animals) Harvey completely revolutionized Galen's concept of circulation. He not only described the contraction of the heart and its pulmonary circulation but explained the role of the veins in returning blood to the heart and the need for valves in maintaining unidirectional blood flow. Harvey is shown in Fig. 1.1 as he appeared at the time of publication of *de mortu cordis*. [1,2]

Today our knowledge of venous disease is equally dependent on an understanding of the anatomy and function of the leg veins. Because many generations of anatomists have redefined the structure and configuration of the venous system there are many different names used to describe the veins of the leg. We use nomenclature generally agreed upon by English-speaking phlebologists. [3] However, because much of the phlebological literature is in German and French their equivalents are provided for clarity.

Special attention is paid to those veins and anatomic features which are frequently associated with venous disease but which may not be adequately described in regular anatomical texts. Also, many anatomic variations are found in the leg's venous system which are not often described in texts.

Configuration of the venous system

If we visualize the vascular system as seen from the skin surface, the first structures are the capillary loops. Lying just beneath the epidermis, the series of loops begin as arterioles which ascend from the deeper dermis. At the top of the loop the tiny vessel becomes a venule. Gas and fluid exchanges occur here as the blood begins its journey back to the heart.

Post-capillary venules measure about 12–30 μm and

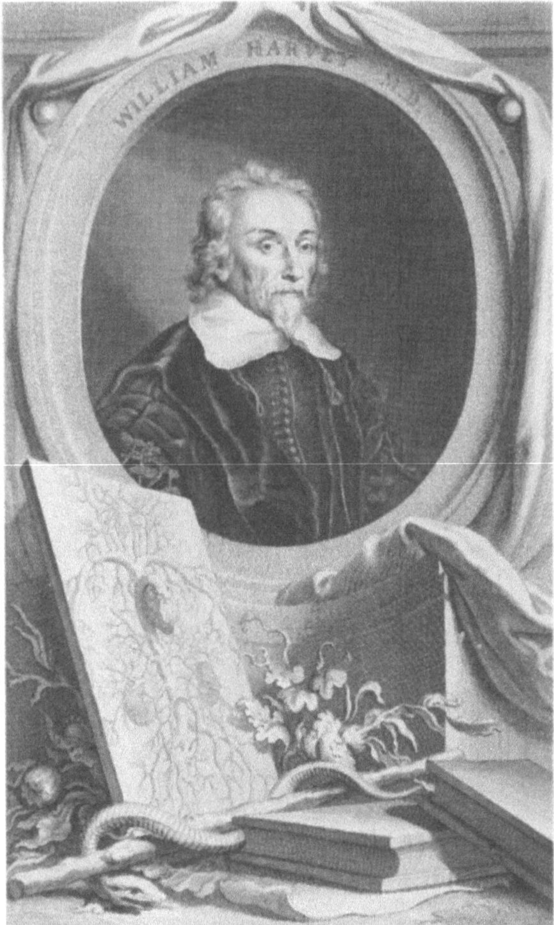

Figure 1.1 William Harvey, M.D. at the time of publication of *de motu cordis* in 1628. Having received his medical degree at the University of Padua, Italy he returned to England to receive an M.D. degree from Cambridge and become a member of the Royal College of Physicians. He entertained a busy clinical practice and lectured at the College of Physicians for 25 years before publishing his famous work. (Used with the kind permission of the Royal Society of Medicine, London.)

run in a horizontal direction as they enlarge and coalesce with other venules. These tiny veins can often be seen in light-skinned people as they run in the deep dermis or subdermis.

As the size of the subcutaneous vein increases to about 1 mm in diameter many are accompanied by small arteries. Still within the subcutaneous fat, the many collecting veins join to direct the blood into one of the saphenous systems.

Within the muscles or other structures of the leg, the same transition of arteriole to venule by way of the capillary network is found. As the veins enlarge they may run outside the muscles or within them as they collect blood from surrounding venules.

Histology

When compared with the structure of arteries, veins appear to be thin-walled and weak. Under normal conditions they prove to be remarkably strong and durable. Like arteries they are composed of three tissue layers, the tunica intima, the tunica media and the tunica adventitia. Veins contain smaller amounts of collagen and muscle and far less elastic tissue than their arterial counterparts and are therefore less resistant to increased pressures. [4]

Intima

Endothelial cells comprise the intimal layer and are supported by a thin basement membrane and an elastic lamina. The endothelium may be no more than one cell thick and represent the major structure of the smallest capillaries. Although the intima seems to be a simple physical structure, it is biologically active and mediates many blood clotting activities. For example endothelial cells produce activators of fibrinolysis in larger quantities than their arterial counterparts. Prostaglandins, especially prostacyclin, are secreted in all veins and have a distinct antiplatelet-aggregating property. These substances are also inhibitors of thromboxane, a powerful platelet aggregator derived from the platelets themselves. Factor VIII is also produced by the endothelium although its venous function is not clearly understood. [5]

Media

As found in medium-sized arteries, the media of veins is formed of muscle fibers arranged in various striae. Their configuration depends on the size and function of the vein. Elastic fibers and connective tissue support and separate the layers, usually three in number. The muscular layers create in the vein the contractility which maintains venous tone.

Adventitia

This outer layer is primarily supportive in function. Its strength is derived from interwoven collagen whose fibers run in different directions. Elastic tissue is prominent in larger veins and permits distensibility necessary to accommodate for changes in venous volume without changing venous pressure. The adventitia is loosely attached to the tissues which surround it. Nourishment is provided to the vein wall by vasovasora which enter through the adventitial layer.

In the normal state the thin-walled construction permits compressibility in response to muscular contraction and at the same time distensibility to compensate for volume changes. On the other hand the fragile make-up and lack of surrounding tissue support render them vulnerable to increased blood volume and venous hypertension.

Many variations are seen in this histologic picture depending on the size, location and function of the particular vein. Changes also are seen in normal veins as they age and with varying stages of venous disease.

Venous innervation

Often forgotten is the fact that veins are liberally supplied with nerves, both sensory and autonomic. Venous tone, which determines the amount of blood in the venous system, is regulated through a complex network of neuroreceptors both central and peripheral. [6]

Many drugs and other external stimuli influence venous tone as well. For example any medical student who has tried to start a difficult intravenous line knows that a vein will dilate if it is warmed or if it is lightly tapped with the finger. Sclerotherapists frequently observe a proximal vein contract tightly when a tiny amount of sclerosant is injected distally. The surgeon who operates under local anesthesia also observes that even varicose veins constrict when bathed in a solution containing epinephrine.

Symptoms associated with venous disease may be related to inflammation, compression or stretching of the tiny nerves caused by the disease process.

Embryology

A knowledge of the basic embryologic changes helps one to understand the many variations found in venous anatomy as well as the congenital phlebologic diseases which one sees occasionally.

Both the arterial and venous systems develop from a primitive capillary network. On the lateral border of the flattened limb bud a primary marginal or fibular vein forms around the 6th week of gestation. It is the original outflow tract for the tiny arterial plexes which

are forming simultaneously in the leg. As the leg develops, the upper portion of the new vein disappears while the caudal portion continues to mature. This original vein system forms both the lesser saphenous vein (LSV) and the anterior tibial veins.

Variations in the disappearance of the upper portion accounts for the wide variations found in the adult LSV. Not only does its attachment to the deep venous system vary considerably but a variety of other venous channels can be found, frequently in the posterior and lateral thigh. [7] A few weeks after the original lateral marginal vein appears, as shown in Fig. 1.2, a secondary marginal vein develops on the medial border of the limb. From this the greater saphenous vein (GSV) arises separately, giving off the femoral and posterior tibial veins as well. This embryologic progression is more orderly and uniform than that of the primary lateral plexus. The resulting anatomy of the greater saphenous, posterior tibial and femoral systems is more constant in configuration.

Venous sytems of the foot

Until recent years the true nature of the feet veins has eluded careful study. The anatomic structures have been well described in the past but the function of the various plexes of veins is just now being understood.

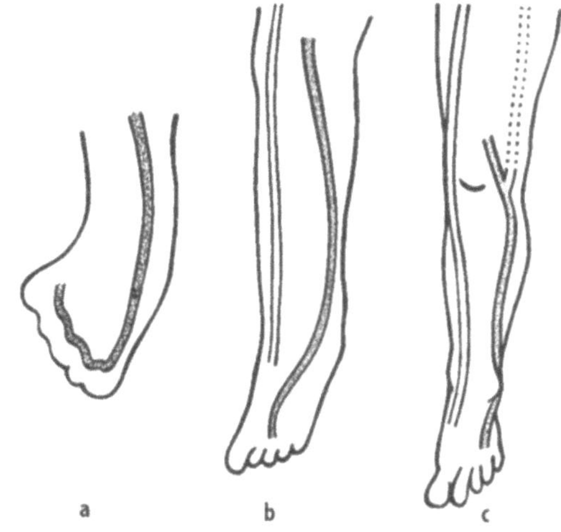

Figure 1.2 The stages of development of the two embryologic vein systems in the leg are shown. **a** A lateral (fibular) marginal vein drains the original primitive arterial plexus. **b** A second marginal vein soon appears and continues to develop on the medial border of the limb forming the greater saphenous and posterior tibial veins. **c** The upper portion of the lateral branch disappears in varying degrees while the residual elements form the lesser saphenous and anterior tibial veins. (Modified and redrawn from Weber J, May R (1990) Funktionelle Phlebologie. Georg Thieme, Stuttgart.)

Superficial dorsal venous arch

Encircling the dorsum of the foot is the *dorsal venous arch*. Because it has no fascial covering and is situated subcutaneously it is prominent and easily identified. A composite vein, it collects blood from both deep and superficial veins of the foot and may exhibit bidirectional flow from each.

The dorsal arch is the mother of the two saphenous systems as seen in Fig. 1.3. A well-formed *medial marginal vein* continues upward as the GSV whereas the lateral limb of the dorsal arch, the *lateral marginal vein*, meanders about, is less visible but eventually forms the LSV. Two other branches, the anterior and posterior arch veins, separate themselves from the dorsal arch to ascend the leg along their own pathways.

Deep plantar venous arch

Each toe has two sets of digital veins, dorsal and plantar. The dorsal digital veins join in the clefts between the toes to form the metatarsal veins which drain into the dorsal venous arch.

The deep plantar venous arch is a triangular group of veins formed by the coalition of deep interdigital and metatarsal veins. The arch, running from the first interosseous space to the base of the fifth metatarsal bone, is made up of a number of coalescing veins which may measure 1 cm or more in diameter. Many smaller twigs and perforating veins drain blood from the muscular veins and the superficial tissues of the sole to the medial and lateral limbs of the arch. The medial and lateral plantar veins finally join beneath the medial malleolus to form the paired posterior tibial veins.

At the first interosseous space a constant large perforating vein joins the deep and superficial venous arches. Like many veins of the plantar arch it is said to be valveless. [8] This connecting vein is the origin of the paired anterior tibial veins, venae comites of the anterior tibial artery. Called the dorsalis pedis artery at this point, the vessels run beneath the taut fascia of the dorsum of the foot and are not visible. At the flexion crease of the ankle they become the anterior tibial artery and veins.

As is true of the superficial arch, blood collected in the deep plantar system has a choice of upward flow by either the deep or superficial system. It may flow to the superficial system by way of the interdigital communicating vein to the dorsal arch vein and then to either of the saphenous systems. If it chooses to remain in the deep system it can flow upward by either the anterior or posterior tibial veins. [9]

This bidirectional flow was thought to be unique to the foot veins but has recently been observed in the perforating veins of the calf as well. The phlebogram shown in Fig. 1.4 illustrates both the deep venous arch and portions of the superficial arch veins.

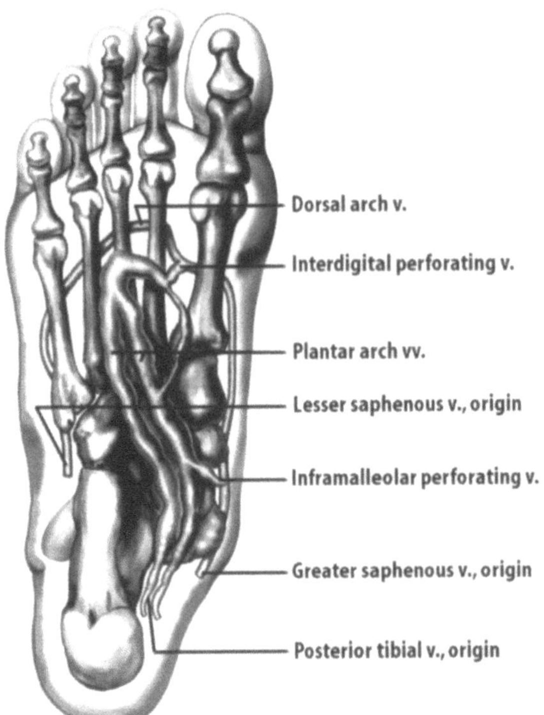

Figure 1.3 This plantar view illustrates the relationship between the deep plantar venous plexus and the superficial dorsal venous arch. The origins of the two saphenous systems are seen as extensions of the medial and lateral branches of the dorsal arch. The valveless interdigital and submalleolar perforating veins permit bidirectional blood flow between the deep and superficial systems. (Modified and used with the kind permission of the Kendall Co.)

Superficial venous system

Most of the varicose veins treated by the phlebologist are derived from this system which resides outside the muscular fascia. When larger varicose veins are present they are usually dilated tributaries of the saphenous vein system.

The saphenous trunks are frequently called the long and short saphenous veins and sometimes the internal and external saphenous veins; in German, *saphena magna* and *saphena parva*. Unlike the deep veins the saphenous vein trunks and branches are not regularly accompanied by arteries.

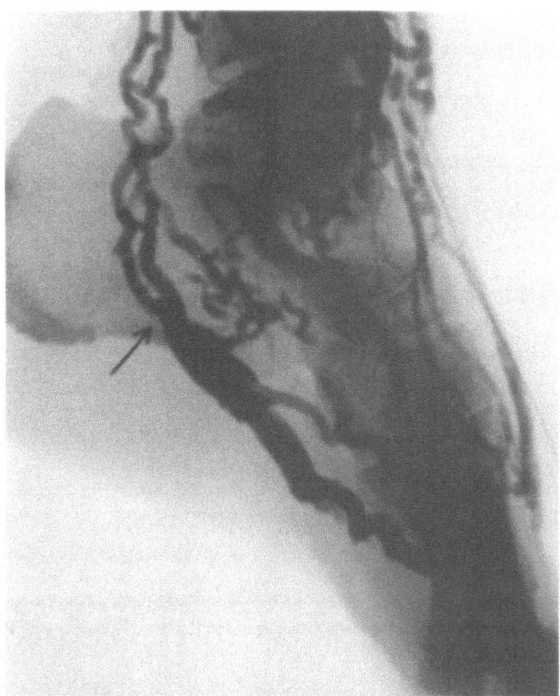

Figure 1.4 The deep venous plexus of the foot is sharply outlined with dye. The arrow marks the beginning of the paired posterior tibial veins as they pass behind the medial malleolus of the tibia to continue upward. The anterior tibial veins are outlined on the dorsum of the foot as well. (Used with the kind permission of Prof. Dr. med. Wolfgang Hach and Springer-Verlag, Heidelberg.)

Large quantities of smooth muscle in their media make the saphenous trunks the strongest veins of the body, a fact which allows them to be used as arterial substitutes.

Greater (long) saphenous vein (GSV)

Taking its origin from the medial limb of the dorsal arch, the GSV runs from the foot to the groin on the inner surface of the leg. As the major superficial collecting and transport vein of the leg, it is also the longest vein in the body. Its accessibility and inherent strength make it a favorite choice for coronary artery bypass and other vascular substitutions.

It is readily seen just in front of the medial malleolus of the tibia only to disappear beneath the superficial fascia a few centimeters above. Because of its superficial and constant position, this has been the traditional site for obtaining venous access by cutdown.

From the ankle the GSV ascends the calf along the border of the gastrocnemius muscle. It is in its most superficial position as it passes over the medial condyles of the tibia and femur. Its course in front of the popliteal crease is far more posterior than one might expect.

It continues an oblique path directly up the thigh on the medial border of the sartorius muscle where it measures 3–5 mm in diameter. As it ascends it is lying directly on the muscular fascia and beneath the superficial fascia. The superficial fascia is a continuation of Scarpa's fascia which develops from the fascia lata. Although a distinct tissue layer, it is thin, surrounded by loose areolar tissue, but apparently provides support for the GSV until it thins out above the knee. [10]

Saphenofemoral junction (SFJ)

Figure 1.5 demonstrates how the GSV in its last 3–4 cm flares out as it curves down to join the femoral vein. The flared GSV often joins the femoral vein flatly, i.e. *en face*. Both the SFJ and the saphenopopliteal junction (SPJ) are called the *crosse* in French, *Krosse* in German. In French, crosse suggests the shape of a bishop's staff or a shepherd's crook, the form the saphenous takes as it curves to join the femoral vein. The racket used in the game of lacrosse is also called a crosse. [11]

Anatomically the SFJ lies in the center of the femoral (Scarpa's) triangle, 2–3 cm lateral to and 2–3 cm inferior to the pubic tubercle. The triangle is formed by the inguinal ligament above, the adductor longus muscle medially, and the sartorius muscle laterally. The femoral triangle is easily demonstrated by flexing and abducting the leg, the frog-leg position, which stretches the muscles leaving the triangle as a depression. When compared with many phlebologic structures, the muscular triangle and venous junction are constant in position.

The vein at this point runs through the *fossa ovalis* (oval window), a funnel-shaped opening in the surrounding cribiform fascia. The fossa ovalis represents the beginning of the femoral canal. [12]

Traditionally the SFJ was identified by palpating the femoral artery then moving one finger-breadth medial. Doppler examination now identifies the SFJ exactly. In clinical practice the junction is usually directly beneath the inguinal skin crease although it may be proximal to the crease in obese patients and below the groin crease in thin people.

SFJ tributaries

There are a number of small tributaries at the SFJ which drain blood from the groin, lateral thigh and pudendal region and enter the saphenous just at the junction or within 1–2 cm. Sometimes they enter the medial or lateral surface of the femoral vein itself. Most anatomy

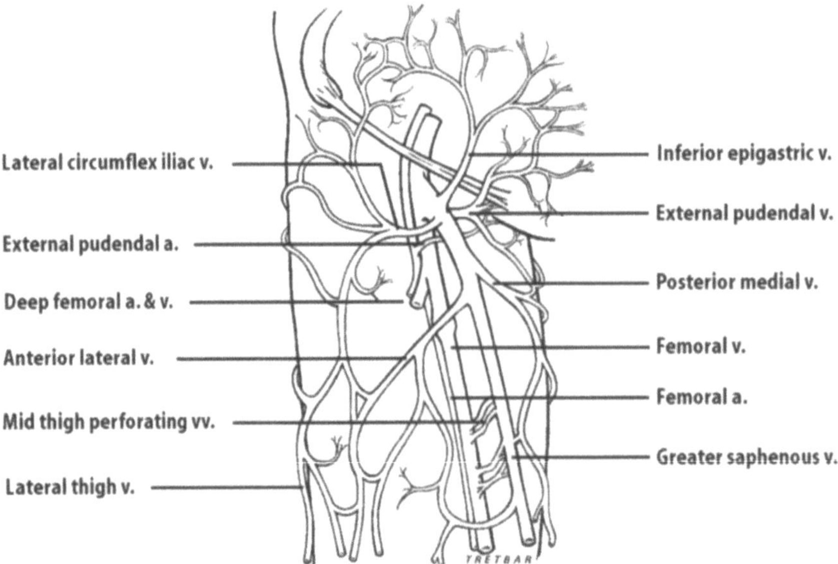

Figure 1.5 The upper thigh exhibits a complex network of tributaries draining into the greater saphenous vein (GSV). The femoral artery and vein are seen passing beneath Poupart's ligament with the saphenofemoral junction positioned a few centimeters below. Mid thigh perforating veins connect the GSV directly with the femoral vein. In life the tributaries show marked variations is size, position and distribution.

books name three separate veins. Surgical dissections by the author show that there is always one tributary and usually three but that there may be as many as six. Most tributaries divide into smaller twigs within 1–2 cm of the entrance into the saphenous. When normal they measure 1–2 mm in diameter but may be as large as the saphenous vein itself. A tiny valve is easily seen just at the junction of the tributary with the saphenous. [4]

Superficial inferior epigastric vein

This tributary drains blood from the lower abdomen and groin areas. It has wide connections with all of the tributaries of the GSV and may not be identifiable as a distinct vein during surgery. On the other hand it may be the first vein encountered during a surgical dissection. It is then quite superficial and can be followed down to the junction.

Superficial external pudendal vein

The scrotum, penis and groin skin in the male and the vulval and perineal areas in women are drained by this vein or veins. It may course over the pubic bone and join the contralateral vein, becoming enlarged with severe pelvic varices or iliac obstruction. It may also become enlarged when varicocoele is present in the male or with vulvopudendal varices in the female.

Superficial lateral circumflex iliac vein

This tributary also drains the lower abdomen as well as the upper and lateral thigh and hip. This too has multiple connections with the many other branches of the saphenous vein. Many of these branching veins are accompanied by small arteries originating from the femoral artery but joining the vein at some distance from the saphenous vein.

An exception is the tiny external pudendal artery which may accompany its vein near the saphenous. In 6% of more than 500 dissections by the author this tiny pudendal artery crosses over the saphenous rather than behind it.

Many illustrations show it as a rather large artery. [13] In fact its true anatomic size and position have not been accurately described before. It is a tiny artery, measuring no more than 1 mm in diameter. It is constant in position when lying beneath the vein. As it runs obliquely upward from the femoral artery it forms the inferior rim of the fossa ovalis.

Because of its size and position it may not be visualized immediately during surgical dissection of the junction and it bleeds vigorously when severed. It should be preserved if possible because it supplies blood to the penis in males and to the vaginal area in females. Its position makes it equally vulnerable to the sclerotherapist who attempts to obliterate the SFJ with injections.

There are deeper analogs of these veins which drain into the femoral vein and which are accompanied by arteries. The best known of the deeper veins is the inferior epigastric vein which, with its artery, forms the medial border of the internal spermatic ring. It then runs upward through the rectus muscle, becoming the superior epigastric vein and finally the internal mammary vein. This entire epigastric system forms one of the major systemic bypasses for vena caval obstruction or in cases of portal hypertension.

GSV thigh branches

Although veins only receive tributaries and do not give off "branches" the use of the word branch to describe the larger tributaries of the saphenous veins is common practice. To this end two large branches join the saphenous trunk in the upper thigh, the anterior lateral thigh vein (anterior accessory saphenous) and the posterior medial thigh vein (posterior accessory saphenous). Duplication of the GSV is reported to occur in 4–25% of limbs studied radiographically. Ultrasonographic examination would suggest the higher degree of occurrence. When duplicated it may join the posterior medial branch.

Anterior lateral vein (lateral accessory saphenous vein)

Joining the GSV anywhere between the crosse and the mid thigh, this vein is a frequent source of varicosis (refer to Chap. 5). Because it is more superficial than the GSV or the posterior medial branch it is easily identified when diseased. When it assumes a position on the front of the thigh it may be erroneously identified as a varicose GSV. It connects freely with the lateral circumflex iliac vein which is also superficial in position.

The anterior lateral branch originates in the reticular veins of the popliteal area or on the lateral knee and thigh. Here it shares attachments with the LSV behind the knee or with the anterior arch vein high on the lateral calf.

Posterior medial vein (medial accessory saphenous vein)

Meeting the GSV in a higher, more constant position than the anterior lateral vein, usually 5–10 cm below the SFJ, the posterior medial vein continues its course beneath the superficial fascia and upon the deeper muscular fascia as it turns toward the posterior thigh. Because it runs at a deeper level than the anterior lateral vein it is seldom seen as varicose, at least at its origins.

As the posterior branch swings posteriorly below the gluteal crease, it has numerous connections with lower, more superficial branches where the varicose state is expressed. However, it may disappear by penetrating the deeper fascia. A common deeper attachment is with the femoropopliteal vein. This anastomosis was first described by Giacomini in 1873. [14] In most cases the femoropopliteal vein is an extension of the LSV and runs beneath the muscular fascia of the posterior thigh. It may in many cases connect both the femoral and gluteal veins.

Patellar vein

This branch (genicular) is a frequent contributor to varicosities around the knee. The vein travels over, above or below the patella and may anastomose with branches of the lateral thigh vein or the anterior arch vein.

A vein in medial thigh may become varicose and descend along the GSV to open more varicosities in the upper calf. It may be an unnamed branch or an accessory saphenous vein. All of these branches intertwine and may not be individually distinguishable.

Calf branches

Just as there are two major branches which join the GSV in the upper thigh, there are two clinically significant branches which join the GSV in the upper calf as seen in Fig. 1.6. They are often varicose as a result of GSV incompetence.

Anterior arch vein (superficial anterior tibial vein)

The anterior arch vein arises from the mid portion of the dorsal venous arch, runs up the shin in a variable fashion and crosses the tibia medially to join the GSV just below the patella. Even in the normal state it is visible as it crosses the tibia. Its course is superficial to the anterior tibial veins to which it is connected by perforating veins. As noted before there are many connections to the veins of the lateral calf and knee.

Posterior arch vein (superficial posterior tibial veins)

As the most posterior branch of the dorsal venous arch, the posterior arch vein turns behind the medial

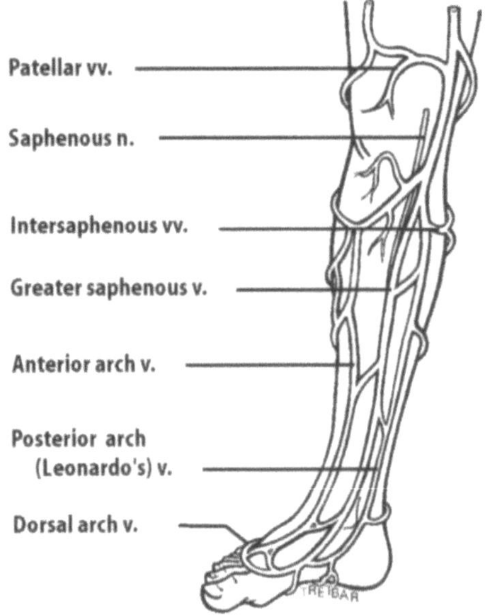

Figure 1.6 The anterior and posterior arch veins are the two major branches of the greater saphenous vein (GSV) in the lower leg. They are interconnected by multiple tributaries and with the lesser saphenous system. As a branch of the femoral nerve the saphenous nerve meets the GSV above the knee and lies next to it in the calf.

malleolus to run up the posterior medial surface of the calf. It too overlies the deeper vein of the same name. Its junction with the GSV is usually lower than that of the anterior arch vein. The vein is seen in some of Leonardo da Vinci's drawings and is sometimes called Leonardo's vein.

Clinically this branch is important because it receives Cockett's perforating veins which are direct connections to the deeper posterior tibial veins. These veins are frequently implicated with cutaneous complications of the ankle and foot.

The posterior arch vein anastomoses freely with the veins of the posterior calf so that drainage may be to either GSV or LSV. An intersaphenous branch is often seen running horizontally in mid calf. These anatomic structures are well delineated in the patient shown in Fig. 5.5.

Lesser (short) saphenous vein (LSV)

Of the two saphenous systems the LSV is less well known or understood because it causes fewer clinical problems. Its early embryological variations have already been described and are of particular significance for the clinician.

In adult life the LSV originates as the lateral limb of the dorsal venous arch, receiving blood from

marginal veins of the sole of the foot as well as sharing branching twigs with the anterior arch vein. It shares drainage with the GSV by way of large intersaphenous bridges on the medial calf and smaller tributaries crossing the Achilles tendon.

From the lateral foot it runs beneath the lateral malleolus, ascends in the groove between the malleolus and Achilles tendon and a few centimeters higher turns to the center of the calf and runs subcutaneously over the tendon.

In mid calf the LSV enters an intrafascial envelope between the bellies of the gastrocnemius muscles, penetrates it in the upper calf where it runs beneath the muscular fascia to enter the popliteal fossa. Its diameter ranges between 3 and 5 mm along its course.

Because of its subfascial position in the upper calf some phlebologists consider the LSV to be a deep vein. Like most we categorize it as a superficial vein. The LSV and its many related surface veins are seen in Fig. 1.7.

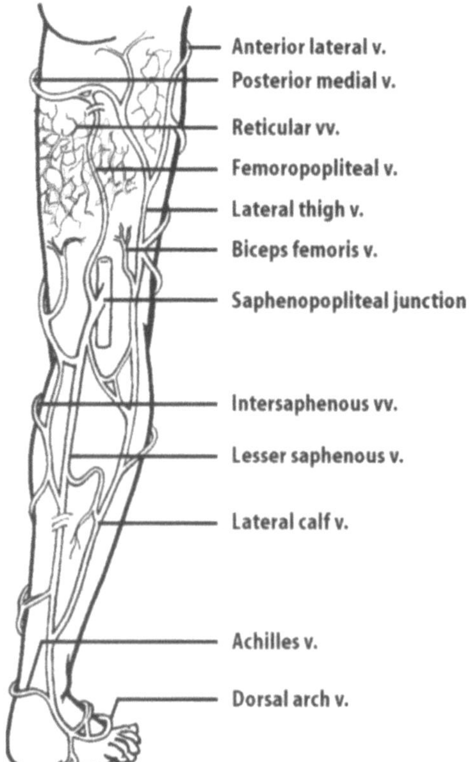

Figure 1.7 This posterior view of the leg demonstrates the many interconnecting veins draining to or from the lesser saphenous vein. Medial surface veins join the two saphenous systems directly. The lateral thigh and calf veins connect the posterior medial and anterior lateral branches of the greater saphenous vein with the femoropopliteal system. Clusters of superficial reticular veins are intimately related to the superficial drainage system.

Saphenopopliteal junction (SPJ)

In a similar fashion to the GSV, the termination of the LSV popliteal vein is called the crosse. In most cases the LSV dips deeply to join the popliteal vein in the vicinity of the popliteal fossa.

Variations in the junction are numerous due to the changes taking place during embryologic development. More than half the time the SPJ is within 5 cm of the flexion skin crease. The rest of the time the crosse may be 5–10 cm above this level.

On occasion, the LSV may not join the popliteal vein at all and continues upward to empty into the gluteal, internal pudendal, femoral vein or the posterior medial branch of the GSV. On rare occasion the LSV may join the deep veins in the calf rather than their conjoined popliteal vein or it may join the GSV itself.

When the SPJ is within the popliteal fossa the gastrocnemius veins may join it or they may join the popliteal vein.

A frequent tributary of the SPJ is the femoropopliteal vein, which runs upward from the junction. Its termination is variable and has been described.

Popliteal fossa

Like the femoral triangle, the boundaries of the popliteal fossa are formed by the edges of the surrounding muscles. The popliteal vein, artery and nerve lie together within the popliteal fossa. Arterial branches supply the assorted muscle groups and overlying skin. These are of particular interest to the sclerotherapist as there are reports of small arteries receiving inadvertent injections resulting in skin and muscle necrosis.

Many sural branches spread out from the fossa to their various destinations. Like the femoral nerve in the groin they provide both muscular as well as sensory innervation. They too can be injured during sclerotherapy or surgical treatment of the LSV. These structures are seen in Fig. 1.8.

LSV branches

Like the GSV there are usually two major branches which connect the upper and lower LSV. Without specific names they are usually referred to as the medial and lateral branches. They are superficial, quite variable in position and perforate the muscular fascia near their junctions with the LSV.

The *popliteal area vein* of Dodd has been described as a specific vein which connects superficial vessels with the popliteal vein at the center of the popliteal fossa. [15]

Lateral calf branch

The lateral branch takes its origins from the LSV at the ankle or from the many small tributaries which

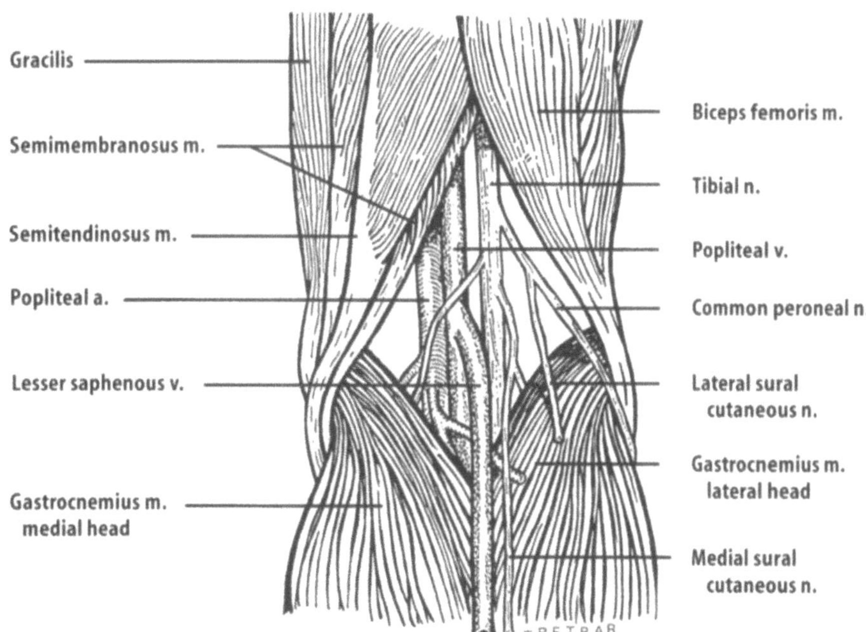

Figure 1.8 This diagram of the right popliteal fossa illustrates the complex network of neurovascular structures with which the phlebologist must work. The sural nerve, often accompanied by a small artery, runs precariously near the lesser saphenous vein in the cleft between the heads of the gastrocnemius muscles. All structures within the fossa vary greatly in position and arrangement.

cross the lateral malleolus from the dorsal venous arch. It wanders up the outer edge of the gastrocnemius muscle along the line of fusion of the deep fascia with the posterior intermuscular septum.

Many twigs from the anterior arch vein or lower segments of the anterior lateral saphenous vein form a network connecting the LSV and GSV on the outside of the leg. Small perforating veins along the course of the intermuscular septum of the gastrocnemius and soleus muscle join the lateral branches with the deep popliteal and peroneal veins.

Medial calf branch

The medial branch is less distinct and constant. It is intertwined with the larger branches which connect GSV and LSV below the knee, especially the posterior arch vein. Small perforating veins join this network with soleal, gastrocnemial and possibly the popliteal vein as well.

Lateral thigh vein

Although not usually named in anatomical texts, it is a common finding and is especially apparent when varicose. The lateral component may be a remnant of the embryologic lateral marginal vein and an upward extension of the lateral calf vein. Its unique position allows it to join the LSV as well as tributaries of the anterior and posterior branches of the GSV.

Varicose lateral thigh vein is commonly the cause of a halo of spider veins in the upper thigh. In this situation it has been called the "lateral subdermic plexus". [16] This author first demonstrated by Doppler that tiny incompetent perforators around the fibular head may be the cause of its incompetence, a fact important to sclerotherapists. [17]

Another common expression of the lateral thigh vein is seen when it joins adjacent reticular veins. When attached to the LSV it may pass upward in the groove formed by the popliteal fossa and the *biceps femoris muscle* to feed a fan-shaped group of spider telangiectasias on the posterior thigh.

Hach describes another perforating vein of some clinical importance in this area. [15] On examination a varicose posterior lateral thigh vein is found to run up the thigh only to disappear below the gluteal fold. A duplex scan visualizes the *Hach perforating vein* connecting the varicose surface veins with the *deep femoral vein*. These changes are demonstrated in Fig. 1.9.

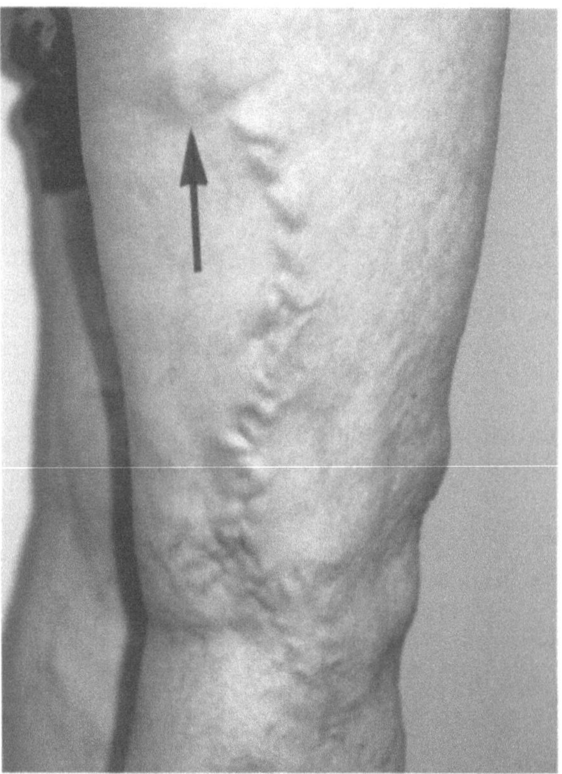

Figure 1.9 This grossly varicose lateral thigh vein originates from the fibular area, ascends the biceps femoris groove to the upper thigh where it disappears. Duplex scanning showed it to descend abruptly to a deep vein. The arrow points to the site of the perforating vein. It was removed by microincisional phlebectomy.

Intersaphenous veins

There are a number of fairly superficial medial branches which join the GSV and LSV below the knee and a few above. Some phlebologists mistakenly call these veins the Giacomini veins. In the normal state blood flows from LSV to GSV. Reversal of flow is common when the GSV is incompetent so that blood refluxes to the LSV. These veins are a frequent site of varicosis. Figure 5.5 shows a markedly dilated intersaphenous vein below an incompetent posterior arch vein.

Reticular vein system

Reticular veins are well known to sclerotherapists but seldom recognized by anatomists. They form a diffuse network of interconnecting veins lying within or just beneath the dermis. When normal they measure 1–2 mm in diameter and are easily seen in light-skinned people forming a patchwork or reticulated pattern.

More prominent on the thighs, they collect blood from smaller tributaries and ultimately drain into one of the saphenous systems. They also drain into non-saphenous veins, such as the system of lateral thigh veins, which in turn empty into the deep system via small perforating veins around the knee.

Because of their color they are usually called "blue veins" although some Canadian phlebologists see them as green. When prominent on the posterior thigh we call them "neighbor veins" or "escalator veins" (they're not visible to the patient, only to the neighbors or to the people behind you on the escalator). Like the larger saphenous tributaries they are valved and direct venous blood upward. Reticular veins are responsible for many of the cosmetic problems of the skin.

Accompanying nerves

As we have seen, the veins are liberally supplied with many tiny nerves. These help regulate venous tone as well as supplying some sense of feeling to the veins. However, larger nerve trunks accompany some of the larger saphenous veins and are of clinical importance when treatment is required.

Accompanying the GSV is the saphenous nerve, a branch of the femoral nerve as seen in Fig. 1.4 and Fig. 7.4. It leaves the adductor canal and approaches the GSV at or just below the knee. Loose areolar tissue attaches it to the vein in the lower half of the leg.

A recognized complication of GSV stripping is injury to the nerve in the lower leg. Nerve damage leaves a numbness on the inner surface of the ankle, for which reason many surgeons strip the GSV only to upper calf.

The LSV is also accompanied by a nerve trunk, the sural nerve. Branches can be found on medial and lateral sides of the vein. They too can be injured by treatment, not only from surgical trauma but from perivenous inflammation following injection sclerotherapy.

Deep venous system

Buried within and between the muscles, the deep veins collect blood from the foot, from the muscles and from the superficial system via the two saphenous junctions and many perforating veins. Conducting veins in the calf form a common larger vein at the knee. This system provides a low pressure conduit for blood to pass out of the lower leg to the pelvis.

Liberally supplied with valves, the deep veins are thinner-walled than the superficial veins but are better supported by the surrounding muscles which themselves are enclosed by a thin, tough and inelastic envelope called *fascia*. Because of its inelasticity, the fascia expands little during muscular contraction. When the muscles contract the veins collapse and expel the contained blood. This action creates the propelling force which returns the blood upward against the pull of gravity. [18]

General configuration

The muscle groups of the leg are arranged into compartments. Major muscle compartments of the leg are the anterior, lateral and superficial and deep posterior compartments. These compartments are further defined by another series of thin fascial envelopes surrounding the individual muscle groups.

Buried within the muscle compartments are two types of deep veins which are of clinical importance: the *intermuscular* veins which run alongside and between muscle groups; and the *intramuscular* veins which lie within the muscles themselves. The general relationships of these veins are demonstrated in Fig. 1.10.

Three groups of intermuscular veins, the *anterior* and *posterior tibial* and the *peroneal*, join in the upper calf to form a common trunk, the *popliteal vein*. Various intramuscular veins, especially those from the *soleus* and *gastrocnemius* muscles, empty their contents into the deep system in the upper calf as well.

As the popliteal vein enters the thigh it turns medially around the femur through a canal made by the adductor muscle (Hunter's canal), and is then called the *superficial femoral vein*. It is joined by the *deep femoral vein* (profundus) a few centimeters above to become the *common femoral vein*. The SFJ lies a few more centimeters above this point. The deep femoral vein itself seldom contributes to the common venous problems of the leg.

The term "superficial femoral" may be confusing since it is a deep vein and not in any way superficial. For example if the superficial femoral vein is subject to thrombophlebitis it is treated as a DVT and not with simpler measures reserved for superficial phlebitis.

At the point beneath the flexion crease of the groin the common femoral vein is joined by the GSV. The femoral vein lies medial to the femoral nerve and artery and passes beneath the inguinal ligament through the femoral canal to enter the pelvis, where it becomes the external iliac vein.

A few cms higher the external iliac vein becomes

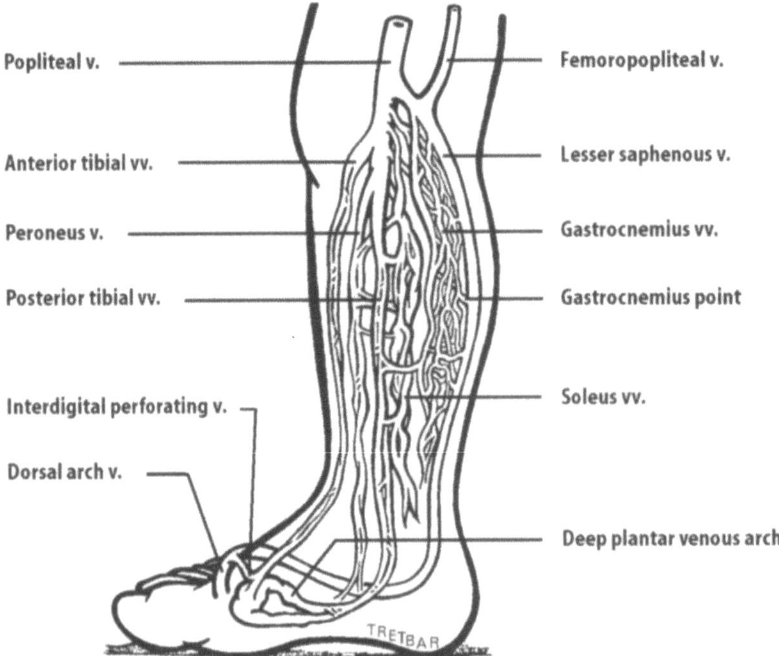

Figure 1.10 The deep venous system of the lower leg is outlined diagrammatically to demonstrate the numerous connections between the muscular and paired intermuscular veins. The origins of the anterior and posterior tibial veins from the plantar arch are clarified.

the common iliac vein by its junction with the internal iliac vein which has ascended from the posterior pelvis. The junction of the contralateral iliac vein creates the inferior vena cave which continues up the trunk ultimately to enter the right heart. [19]

Intermuscular veins (venae comites)

Below the knee the intermuscular veins are paired as they run alongside the artery and are termed *venae comites*. They derive their names from the artery which they accompany and anastomose freely with adjoining muscular and perforating veins.

Three major groups of intermuscular veins are identified in the calf, the *posterior tibial*, the *anterior tibial*, and the *peroneal veins*. Since they run in a vertical position they are generically called axial veins.

Because of their tubular shape they are called "stem veins" by some British phlebologists. This term is confusing since the word *stem* is used by German-speaking phlebologists to describe the saphenous trunks. Stem is a cognate for the German word *Stamm* which means trunk or stem. Its probably best to avoid all of these confusing terms. [7]

Posterior tibial veins

In the ankle the pulse of the posterior tibial artery behind the medial malleolus marks the beginning of the posterior tibial veins. As this point the veins are already paired and drain the deep medial and lateral plantar veins and those surface veins not joining the long saphenous.

The posterior tibial veins run up the back of the leg in the deeper portion of the posterior compartment. In the subcutaneous tissue immediately above them is the posterior arch vein (superficial posterior tibial vein). The superficial and deep posterior tibial venous systems are joined together by Cockett's and Sherman's perforating veins. [20–22]

Anterior tibial veins

This paired deep vein originates from the valveless communicating vein which connects the deep venous arch with the superficial dorsal arch in the first inter-metatarsal space. It is accompanied by the anterior tibial artery which on the dorsum of the foot is known as the dorsalis pedis artery.

Pulses of both anterior and posterior arteries are palpable in the normal individual with the dorsalis pedis being more variable in position and somewhat weaker. From its origin on the dorsum of the foot the vascular bundle runs up the anterior compartment lateral to the tibia. The bundle lies on the interosseous membrane which connects the tibia and fibula. At the junction of the two bones at the knee the vessels penetrate the fascia to join the upper limits of the posterior tibial vein in the popliteal space.

As is true of the posterior veins, the anterior tibial veins are accompanied in the superficial position by the anterior arch vein (superficial anterior tibial vein). Small crural perforating veins join the two venous systems as well.

Peroneus vein

Radiographically the peroneal vein arises from the most lateral region of the heel and appears between or behind the tibia and fibula. Generally it is single and rarely paired as is the case with the other calf veins. Here it drains the posterior and lateral muscular compartments along with the posterior tibial veins.

The peroneal veins merge with the posterior tibials in the upper calf to form a common trunk, the tibioperoneal vein. Some anatomists consider the peroneal to be only a large tributary of the posterior tibial vein.

In the usual situation the anterior tibial trunk joins the tibioperoneal trunk below the popliteal crease. One of the anatomic variations in this region is a high junction of the anterior tibial branch 5–10 cm above the crease. On a phlebogram or ultrasonography this variation has the appearance of a doubled popliteal vein.

Intramuscular veins

As previously mentioned, the intramuscular veins are those which run inside the muscle itself, collecting blood from the muscle fibers. Of the many muscular veins only two are of general clinical importance, the gastrocnemius and the soleus. Their respective muscles surround the back of the calf and flex Achilles tendon. Contraction of these two muscle groups during walking generates marked pressure within the veins and is responsible for most of the pumping action of the calf.

Soleus veins

The soleal veins are often sinusoidal, i.e. without specific form, and may be valveless. They drain into

the peroneal vein through a number of trunks and may have connections with the posterior tibial veins. They communicate with the superficial venous system through perforating veins, especially at the soleus point (German: punkt) on the upper medial calf. Many connections are made with the LSV and its tributaries.

Gastrocnemius veins

The gastrocnemial veins are usually straighter and thinner and contain more valves than the soleal veins. A phlebogram will show as many as 10–15 collecting tributaries in each head which ultimately form a common trunk, which in turn drains into the popliteal vein. At the time of surgery small tributaries are often found entering the LSV as well.

The *gastrocnemius point* marks the attachment of Achilles tendon to the two heads of the gastrocnemius muscles in mid calf. *May's perforating vein* joins the gastrocnemius veins with the LSV at approximately this point. [15]

Like the soleus veins the gastrocnemius may undergo regressive changes and appear fusiform or sinusoidal on phlebography. They are difficult to evaluate with ultrasonography.

Anatomical variations in this area may be as high as 50%, creating problems for the examiner. Evaluation of varicose problems in the calf must therefore be extremely thorough to determine which vein is responsible for the venous incompetence.

Femoropopliteal vein

When present it is a tributary of the LSV originating at the SPJ. As an embryologic product of the lateral marginal vein, it, like the LSV itself, may have a variable termination. It runs up the posterior thigh in the subfascial position where, as a deep vein, it may join the femoral or gluteal vein or it can penetrate the muscular fascial to become superficial. Here it may join the posterior thigh vein or the posterior medial branch of the GSV as it loops around the medial thigh.

In most cases blood flow is upward toward the GSV. However, depending on its higher junction there may be downward flow to the lesser saphenous system. In this case an otherwise normal flow might be considered as reflux. Careful evaluation is required to make this determination.

Giacomini's vein

In the late 19th century Giacomini described an anastomosis between veins which, when present, lay subfascially in the posterior thigh. [14] The anastomosis connected a vein originating from the LSV (? femoropopliteal vein) to a posterior medial vein originating from the GSV (? posterior medial vein). This connection can be seen in Fig. 1.7.

Perforating veins

Perforating veins receive their descriptive title from the fact that they perforate or penetrate the fascia of the muscular compartments. They connect superficial and deep veins at points other than the saphenous junctions. Perforating veins are valved, usually with the valves appearing in the subfascial position. As with the remainder of the venous system blood flow is usually from superficial to deep vein or upward toward the heart.

Perforating veins are frequently called communicating veins by English phlebologists. To avoid confusion we stick with the term perforating vein or simply perforator. We designate communicating veins as those which connect veins of the same system. [22]

When visualized radiographically the perforators are usually double, measure 1–2 mm in diameter and run in an upward direction from their superficial vein as shown in Fig. 4.15. Hach says that when measured they always enter the deep vein at an angle of less than 60 degrees.

GSV perforators

Clinically significant perforating veins along the GSV trunk occur in the thigh and just above and below the knee. The branches and tributaries of the saphenous trunks are also studded with perforating veins. Many are located along intermuscular septa where the veins perforate the fascia.

In the upper thigh a few perforators join the anterior lateral and posterior medial saphenous branches to the femoral and gluteal veins. These are of little clinical significance.

For some reason many of the major perforating veins have eponyms rather than proper anatomic names as seen in Fig. 1.11. [18] In the thigh the major perforating veins join the GSV with the superficial femoral vein. The most constantly observed perforators are in mid to lower thigh above the adductor (Hunter's) canal. The adductor canal is the place where the femoral vessels and nerves pass beneath the adductor muscles to turn around the femur from a more superficial position above, to assume a posterior position at the knee. [22, 23]

Usually there are 3–5 perforating veins here. Formerly called adductor perforators, they are more recently termed *Dodd's group*. The middle vein is more constant in position and lies at the lower third of the thigh. The vein at the level of the adductor canal is still called *Hunter's perforator*.

An even lower perforator lies just above the femoral condyle. Often this lower perforator is referred to solely as *Dodd's perforating vein*. This vein may actually pass through the sartorius or adductor muscle.

A hand's breadth below the knee is *Boyd's perforating vein* which joins the GSV with the posterior tibial vein. In lies near the junction of the GSV with the anterior and posterior arch veins and may join either of these two veins as well. When incompetent these paracondylar perforators may be isolated sources of varicose veins.

Three fairly constant perforators sit along the length of the anterior arch vein, connecting it with the deep anterior tibial vein. Also called the *mid crural veins*, the highest is at the edge of the tibia where the arch vein crosses the bone. [15] Smaller perforators in this area join the anterior tibial vessels with the fibular and peroneal veins. These in turn may be joined to the lateral thigh veins and lower extensions of the superficial thigh veins which join the LSV.

Standing in a row above the medial malleolus (Linton's line) are Cockett's perforating veins connecting the posterior arch vein with the posterior tibial veins. Originally studied by Linton and Sherman but later named after Cockett, they are described as being about 6, 12 and 18 cm above the sole of the heel and 1–3 cm behind the tibia. Another perforator may be present 6 cm above this position and is named after Sherman. [24] Current measurements are taken from the medial malleolus in hopes of providing more precise anatomic information to the surgeon.

The lowest of the three Cockett's veins is adjacent to the medial malleolus. It connects the posterior tibial veins with the GSV or its tributaries and is the least problematic for the clinician.

The upper "two" veins are actually groups of tiny paired veins and are clinically more significant than the lower group. They join the posterior arch vein with the posterior tibial veins and sometimes give branches to the GSV.

Competence of the entire perforating vein system is necessary to protect the superficial venous system from the enormous pressure generated by the foot and calf muscle pumps.

Incompetence of low perforating veins, especially when secondary to DVT, is associated with the typical cutaneous complications of chronic venous insufficiency (CVI).

For the surgeon it is important to understand this special anatomy. Stripping the GSV does not necessarily detach these perforators since they are usually

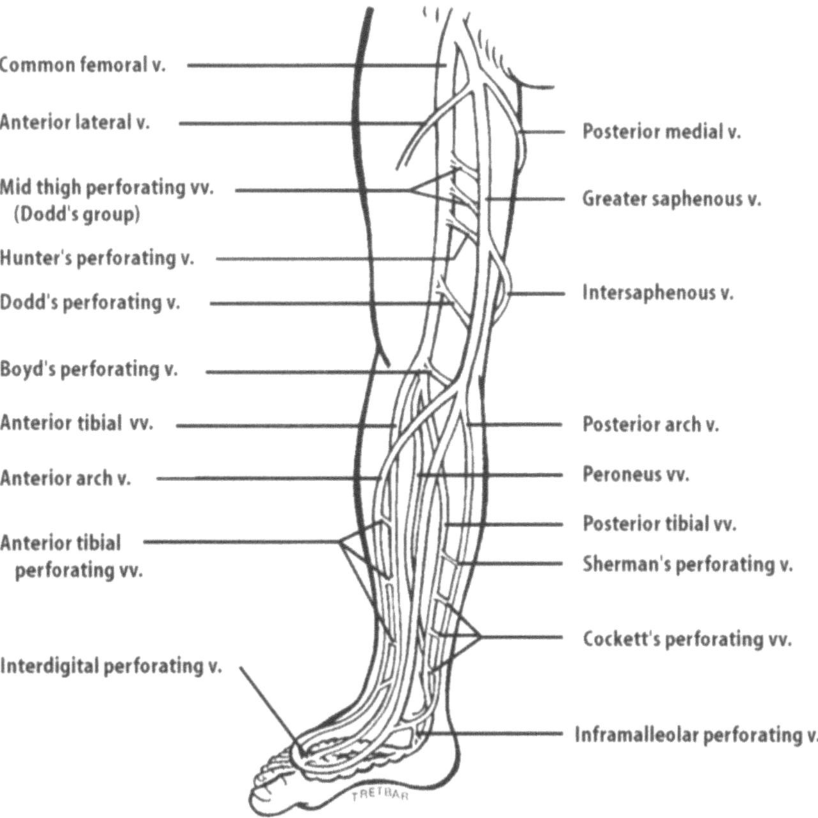

Figure 1.11 Outlined here are the major perforating veins which join the superficial and deep veins. Those of the thigh connect directly to the greater saphenous vein (GSV) whereas those of the posterior tibial vein connect directly to the posterior arch vein and only indirectly to the GSV. Many other perforating veins exist but are not clinically important.

connected to the posterior arch vein and not directly or exclusively to the GSV. For this reason GSV stripping may not be beneficial in the healing of venous ulcers. [19]

Calf perforators

Although the perforating veins of the anterior and medial leg receive a large amount of attention there are many other perforators associated with both groups of deep calf veins.

The well-known gastrocnemius and soleus points represent the sites of their respective muscle perforating veins. Their origins and destinations are more variable than those of the medial leg. The gastrocnemius perforator, already described as May's, is perhaps the most reliably placed. It may be apparent joining the LSV with the gastrocnemius just above the attachment of the Achilles tendon. It may also attach itself to a medial saphenosaphenous vein.

Although there are many small intermuscular connecting veins, the major soleus perforating vein appears in the upper medial calf. It may join the upper posterior arch vein or other branches of the GSV. Many of these joining veins are shown in Fig. 1.12.

The lateral calf perforating veins cause fewer problems than their medial counterparts and are therefore less well known.

Bassi's vein may join the peroneal veins with the LSV or its lateral branches.

Higher on the calf the peroneal veins may join the lateral calf vein near the fibular head, the so-called fibular perforators. As has been noted this set of perforating veins may become incompetent and cause reflux up the lateral thigh or biceps vein. This in turn may be the cause of the fan of lateral thigh telangiectasia or the varicosities of the superficial posterior lateral thigh veins.

The *profunda perforating vein* of Hach has already been described in the upper posterior thigh.

Foot perforators

In the foot many perforating veins do not have valves. In this valveless situation blood can flow in either

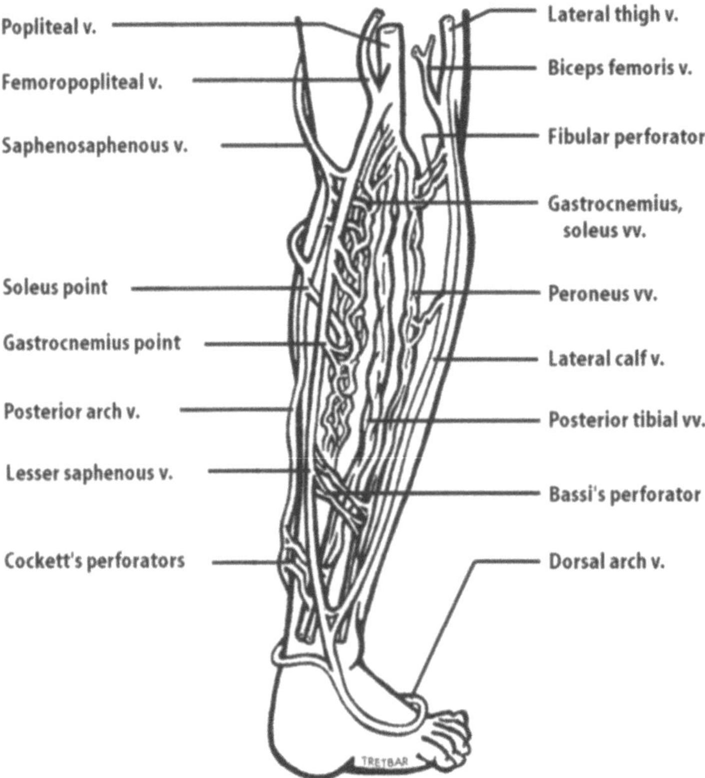

Figure 1.12 The major perforating veins of the lesser saphenous system are shown in a simplified form. For clarity the gastrocnemius and soleus veins are shown as a single unit although they each have separate perforating veins directed to surface veins. The lateral calf and thigh veins are connected primarily to the peroneal veins and may be a cause of surface varicosities.

direction. Much of the flow is from deep to superficial, contrary to the usual direction through perforating veins. Doppler testing, however, shows vigorous flow up the posterior tibial vein when one squeezes the plantar surface.

One such valveless vein has already been described and is found in the first interdigital cleft and connects the deep and superficial venous arches of the foot.

Of the many small perforating veins found along the marginal foot veins, only two are clinically significant. They were described by Kuster and are found beneath both medial and lateral malleoli. [25,26] Isolated varicose veins on the foot may be due to incompetence in any of these perforators since they connect with the deep venous arch which generates an enormous pressure during walking and jumping. [24]

Valves

The health of the venous system is directly related to the health of its valves. Chronic venous disease, in some fashion, is the result of valvular dysfunction.

Healthy valves maintain blood flow toward the heart and prevent reflux; unhealthy valves allow reflux of blood to occur when the person is in the upright position and during exercise.

Valvular embryology

Although the veins reach their adult form of development at about 3 months gestation it is another 2 months before a substantial number of valves can be distinguished. Usually five stages of development are described.

A bulging of the intima is the first sign of a developing valve. As the endothelial structure elongates the vein wall above starts to bulge. The venous wall then thins at the base or sinus of the valve, mostly by loss of circular muscle. When the thickened valve cusp finally thins out the valve becomes functional as shown in Fig. 1.13.

Parietal valves

Those valves encountered most frequently are called parietal valves (German: *Taschenkloppen* = pocket

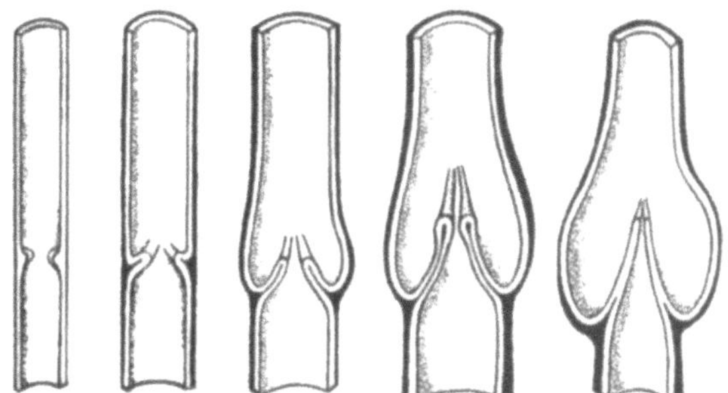

Figure 1.13 This drawing shows the stages in the embryologic development of a typical bicuspid venous valve. The changes represent a continuous folding in of the vein wall so that similar histologic tissues are represented in each portion of the structure. Note that the wall is thinnest at the level of the sinus, a feature which may assist in valve closure. (Modified and redrawn from Weber J, May R (1990) Funktionelle Phlebologie. Georg Thieme, Stuttgart.)

valves). Most venous valves are bicuspid in structure although tricuspid valves are reported. They are usually found along the course of the larger trunk veins and at the termination of a smaller vein as it enters a larger vein. Typical parietal valves are found at the SFJ and SPJ. [27]

At the valve site the vein is somewhat elliptical in shape. The valves are so arranged that the valve cusps are tangential, i.e. parallel, to the skin surface. Pressure from the skin surface or from muscle expansion tends to close or compress the valve cusps. [28]

Structurally the valve consists of the *cusp* (leaflet) which is attached to the vein wall by the *agger*. The varying projections of the valve leaflet form the *cornu*, the *commissure* and the *sinus*.

When looking at the cusp from the lumen of the vein it assumes a horseshoe or crescent shape. Although delicate in appearance it consists of a skeleton of tough collagenous fibers covered with a single layer of endothelial cells. A portion of the collagenous fibers continue into the vein wall and interdigitate with fibers from the opposite valve.

The luminal side of the valve is smooth, formed by a thin elastic layer which lies beneath the luminal endothelium as an extension of the vein's elastic lamina. On the sinus-side of the cusp the endothelial cells form crypts and crevices creating an irregular appearance when viewed microscopically. This may be due to the absence of the thin elastic layer found beneath the luminal endothelium.

The free edge of the cusp is often described as beaded or nodular, although this may have no significance. The tissue which attaches the bottom edge to the vein wall is called the valvular agger, within which can be found a few smooth muscle cells as well as collagen.

As the free and attached edges of the cusp come together near the vein wall they have the appearance

of a horn, the cornu. The junction of the opposing cornua creates a commissure.

The space between the valve wall and the vein wall is called the sinus or pocket. The vein wall adjacent to the sinus is especially thin when compared to other portions of the vein.

Closure of the valve has traditionally been thought to be a simple mechanical action. It was thought that the reversal of blood flow caused the valve cusps to bellow like a parachute occluding the vein lumen and preventing reflux. Although a minute amount of reflux is necessary to initiate closure, recent findings suggest that the valve cusp may play an active role. [29]

Some investigators report that thin neuromuscular fibers can be found running from the agger into the valve cusp. Although their functional significance is questionable, these findings suggest that valve closure may be more than a passive response to the reversal of blood flow. Certainly phlebography and real-time ultrasonography show a complex series of events in the closing response. Refluxing blood can be seen initiating cusp movement. Valve sinus distention then separates the valvular commissures and the cusp edges are tightened. The gross structural elements of a valve are shown in Fig. 1.14.

Ostial valves

Ostial valves are those found at the entry point of a small vein into a much larger vein. These small valves tend to vary in structure and configuration when compared to the parietal valve, which is more regular in structure. For example there is a decrease or absence of agger in many of the tiny valves. There may be only one cusp or a cusp may protrude into the lumen of

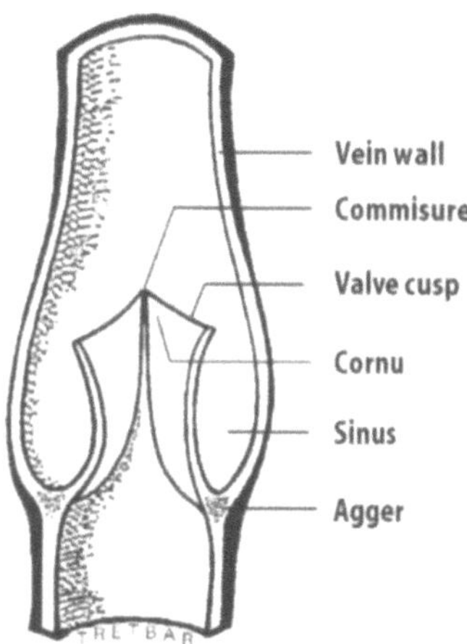

Figure 1.14 The features of a typical adult bicuspid valve. The cusps are relatively thinner than shown but tough enough to withstand the hydrostatic pressure within the veins.

the larger vein. Tiny valves of this type may appear in veins as small as 1 mm in diameter. They are readily apparent in tributaries at the SFJ.

This terminology is confusing as we often call the valve at the opening into a larger vein the ostial valve. The valve at the SFJ is called the ostial valve, sometimes "terminal" valve. When a second valve is present a few cms distal it is called the pre-ostial or "pre-terminal" valve.

Valvular distribution

In general the number of valves increases the more distal the vein. The calf veins for example have valves almost every 2 cm. From a functional viewpoint these numerous valves are better able to distribute the force generated by the contraction of the calf muscles and the hydrostatic pressure from the erect position.

As mentioned earlier, there may be few or no valves in the communicating veins of the foot. This arrangement allows bidirectional flow, the importance of which is still under scrutiny.

The intramuscular muscles of the lower leg are liberally supplied with bicuspid valves of the parietal type. Although the sinusoidal veins of the soleal muscles may be valveless the efferent drainage veins are well valved. Gastrocnemius veins are the other major muscular veins and are liberally supplied with valves, as are their efferent veins.

Two valves usually are found in the popliteal vein of the knee. These are of particular importance. Proper function of the calf muscle pump depends on their competence. [30]

A valve is present in 90% of femoral veins just distal to their junction with the deep femoral vein. There is an irregular distribution of valves above this point.

Both GSV and LSV contain between eight and ten valves. There is always a valve at the termination of the GSV with the femoral vein and usually another one or two valves 3–5 cm distal to it. These valves are of primary importance in the prevention of reflux down the GSV.

There has been considerable attention given to the valves which may or may not be present in the iliofemoral veins above the SFJ. The significance lies in the commonly held view that the long saphenous vein is protected by valves above its juncture with the femoral vein. It is said that the absence of valves in the iliac vein renders the GSV susceptible to the extremes in pressure found in the inferior vena cava and iliac veins.

Although the estimates vary according to author, it is safe to say that there is at least one valve above the SFJ in 35–80% of all limbs. However, valves are rarely found in the common iliac vein. Some studies show that 25% of right common femoral veins are valveless and that as many as 75% of left common femoral veins may be valveless. These data have been used to support the theory of descending valvular incompetence. [31]

Some data suggest that there are more varicose veins in the left leg than right. Consideration is given to the above information and to the fact that the left iliac artery crosses the vein and may impede venous flow from the left leg.

Perforating veins all seem to possess valves except in the foot. Some have up to five valves but two or three are the rule. Most are subfascial in position although some can be found above the muscular fascia. When there is a single valve it is positioned in the perforator just before it enters the deep vein. These valves usually maintain the direction of blood flow from superficial to deep veins.

Comments

The anatomic distribution of veins in the legs is varied and complex. The veins represent a diverse system which collects the blood from a multitude of tiny veins, finally coalescing into single large veins which enter the pelvis.

Contemporary evaluation methods, especially non-invasive testing, have given us a new insight into the anatomic and functional status of the venous systems. In this way we are better able to assess pathologic changes and develop better treatment methods.

References

1. Major RH (1954) History of Medicine, vol. 1. Charles C Thomas, Springfield
2. Laufman H (1986) The Veins. RG Landes, Austin
3. Venous Consensus Conference (Feb 1994) Maui, Hawaii
4. William PL ed (1995) Gray's Anatomy, 38th edn. Churchill Livingstone, London
5. Browse NL, Burnand KG, Lea Thomas M (1988) Diseases of the Veins: Pathology, Diagnosis and Treatment. Edward Arnold, London
6. Netter FH (1990) Atlas of Human Anatomy. Ciba–Geigy, Summit, NJ
7. Weber J, May RF (1990) Funktionelle Phlebologie. Georg Thieme, Stuttgart
8. Lofgren EP, Myers TT, Lofgren KA (1968) The venous valves of the foot and ankle. Surg Gynecol Obstet 127:289–291
9. Gardner AMN, Fox RH (1993) The Return of Blood to the Heart, 2nd rev edn. John Libbey, London
10. Kupinski AM, Evans SM et al (1993) Ultrasonographic characterization of the saphenous vein. Cardiovasc Surg 1:513–517

11. Vigoni M (1983) Phlebologie, les précis pratiques. Maloine, Paris

12. Callander CL (1939) Surgical Anatomy, 2nd edn. WB Saunders, Philadelphia

13. Goldman MP (1995) Sclerotherapy: Treatment of Varicose and Telangiectatic Leg Veins, 2nd edn. Mosby, St Louis

14. Giacomini C (1873) Osservazioni anatomische per servire allo studio della circulazione venosa dell estremita inferiore. Parte I–III. Giornale R Acad Med 1:109. Torino

15. Hach W, Hach-Wunderle V (1997) Phlebography and Sonography of the Veins. Springer, Heidelberg

16. Albanese AR, Albanese AM, Albanese EF (1969) The lateral subdermic venous system of the legs. Vasc Surg 3:81–89

17. Tretbar LL (1989) The origin of reflux in incompetent blue reticular/telangiectasia veins. In Phlebologie '89, Davy A, Stemmer R eds. John Libbey/Eurotext, London/Paris

18. Dodd H, Cockett FB (1976) The Pathology and Surgery of the Veins of the Lower Limb. Churchill Livingstone, Edinburgh

19. Tretbar LL (1995) Deep veins. Dermatol Surg 21:47–51

20. Hobbs JT ed (1977) The Treatment of Venous Disorders. JB Lippincott, Philadelphia

21. Linton RR (1938) The communicating veins of the lower leg and the operative technique for their ligation. Ann Surg 107:582–593

22. Dodd H (1959) The varicose tributaries of the superficial femoral vein passing into Hunter's canal. Postgrad Med J 35:18–22

23. Papadakis K, Christodoulou C, Hobbs J et al (1989) Number and anatomical distribution of incompetent thigh perforating veins. Br J Surg 76:581–584

24. Sherman RS (1949) Varicose veins: further findings based on anatomic and surgical dissections. Ann Surg 130:218–232

25. Kuster S, Lofgren EF, Hollinshead WH (1981) Anatomy of the veins of the foot. Surg Gynecol Obstet 127:187–184

26. May R, Nissl R (1981) Nomenclature of the surgically important connecting veins. In Perforating Veins, May R, Partch H, Staubesand J eds. Urban and Schwarzenburg, München

27. Gottlob R, May R (1986) Venous Valves. Springer, Wien

28. Edwards RJ (1936) The orientation of venous valves in relation to body surfaces. Anat Rec 64:369–377

29. Rose S (1986) Some thoughts on the aetiology of varicose veins. J Cardiovasc Surg 27:534–543

30. Kappert A (1989) Lehrbuch und Atlas der Angiologie. Hans Huber, Bern

31. Basmajian JV (1952) The distribution of valves in the femoral, external iliac and common iliac veins and their relationship to varicose veins. Surg Gynecol Obstet 95:537–542

CHAPTER 2

Venous Function, Dysfunction and Venous Insufficiency

Although the function of the leg veins might seem to be the passive transport of blood from the foot to the heart, the venous system is far more hemodynamically active than the arterial system. In addition to transporting blood back to the heart, the veins are responsible for the regulation of body temperature, balancing cardiac output and as a reservoir for blood. In fact as much as two-thirds of the body's total blood volume may be in the venous system at any one time.

These complex functions depend upon the vein's unique ability to expand and contract, an attribute of its thin-walled construction. This inherent elasticity provides one of the venous system's most important functions, the ability to accommodate to large changes in blood volume with little change in pressure.

Return of blood to the heart

In the normal leg blood is returned to the heart by a number of forces, *vis a tergo* (left ventricular contraction), position, changes in intrathoracic and intra-abdominal pressures and muscular contractions in the legs. Some believe that the sucking action of right atrial contraction, *vis a fonte*, assists in the upward flow of blood to the heart. Proper return of blood depends not only on these factors but on normal valvular function and on adequate refilling of the various pumps.

Foot muscle pump

Often unappreciated is the active role that the foot plays in the return of blood to the heart. In the past it was thought that the return of blood from the foot was primarily a passive event. Weight bearing and contraction of the plantar muscles were thought to transfer blood from the deep venous plexus into the superficial foot veins through valveless perforating veins. Some blood was thought to pass into the deep system to prime it for calf muscle contraction whereas most of the foot's blood passed up the superficial veins.

Using video-phlebography (continuous video imaging during injection of contrast medium), recent studies show a differing series of events. [1] These anatomic and physiologic studies demonstrate that the foot pump is made up of the deep plantar arch, the analog of the superficial dorsal arch, with medial and lateral branches. Here the plantar veins are strung between the anterior and posterior osseous arches like "bow strings". Weight bearing flattens the arch, literally stretching the veins and expelling the blood. During video-angiography, contrary to expectation, weight bearing expelled the dye from the plantar arch veins primarily into the deep, not superficial veins. Blood flow was not induced by contraction of the foot muscles as it is in other pumps of the leg but by the stretching of the veins. Gardner reported that contraction of the pump was powerful enough to overcome a tourniquet pressure of 100 mmHg in the calf.

As discussed in Chap. 1, the arches converge beneath the medial malleolus and form the paired posterior tibial veins, venae comites of the posterior tibial artery. [2] A valveless perforating vein between the first and second metatarsals connects the deep venous arch to another set of deep veins, the dorsalis pedis (anterior tibial) veins (see Fig. 1.3). Most of the small perforating veins in the foot are said to be valveless. The traditional concept has been that blood flows from superficial to deep. However, the very act of weight bearing may prevent flow in this direction. The tension created within the plantar aponeurosis may close the perforating veins and direct blood into the deep system.

In general, flow from the foot may proceed from the plantar plexus up the deep veins, i.e. anterior and posterior tibial, or into the saphenous systems. Gardner suggests that the channel selected for flow depends on a number of factors: position of the foot, temperature, volume of blood contained in either deep or superficial system and the state of muscular contraction in the calf.

Doppler examination of the foot confirms the flow of blood from the foot into both deep and superficial veins. When a Doppler probe is placed over the posterior tibial vein and the foot squeezed, marked flow is heard. There is usually flow heard over the saphenous trunks as well.

Figure 2.1 shows in diagrammatic form the configuration of the foot and muscle pumps and the outflow pattern resulting from activation of the foot pump. Our laboratory has been particularly interested in the function of the foot pump. We have found air plethysmography (APG) to be a useful method of evaluating exercise-induced blood flow. APG studies have traditionally been used to measure the global function of venous blood flow at the level of the calf. These data naturally include the activity of both foot and calf pumps (see Fig. 4.13).

Our problem was to isolate the function of the foot pump from that of the calf muscle pump and if possible to determine the amount of blood expelled into the deep and superficial systems. To do this a system was devised which combines APG and quantified Doppler flow.

Initially a traditional APG examination was performed using tiptoeing as the exercise form. This exercise activates both calf and foot muscle pumps, the sum of which is recorded in the usual fashion.

To isolate the function of the foot pump from that of the calf muscle pump, the leg and foot were then immobilized so that the calf muscles were inactive. The system was designed so that the APG measuring cuff was not disturbed and the saphenous veins were not occluded.

While the patient was standing the immobile leg was raised and then pressed onto the floor, as if walking stiff-legged. "Clumping", as we call it, was continued at 1 s intervals for 10 s. This method of exercise compressed the foot pump without activating the calf muscles.

The reading obtained from the clumping represented the outflow from the foot pump into the calf and thigh. The contribution of the calf pump was calculated by subtracting this value from the original reading.

A group of volunteers, mostly operating room nurses without demonstrable venous disease, were tested in this manner. Although the findings were not analyzed statistically the results were consistent enough to provide some interesting information about the pumping action of the two muscle groups.

The major surprise was that in many examinations the foot pump contributed almost half of the blood leaving the calf. To determine the amount of blood

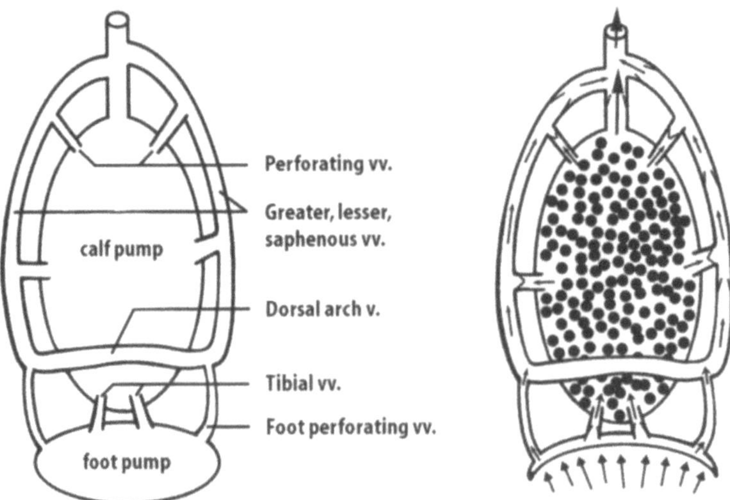

Figure 2.1 (Left) The leg at rest with the veins filled. The foot pump is represented at the base with outflow through the anterior and posterior tibial veins. The foot perforators may also act as outflow. The calf pump has inflow via the tibials and the perforating veins from the two saphenous systems. (Right) The foot pump has been compressed and its blood expelled. The tibial veins fill directly into the calf compartments whereas the foot perforating veins fill the saphenous systems resulting in some outflow.

moving up the GSV a flat Doppler probe was attached with Velcro over the GSV just above the knee. This permitted a continuous monitoring of flow velocity during exercise, whether by tiptoeing or clumping.

The cross-sectional area of the vein was measured sonographically and the flow quantified by multiplying area by velocity. Flow through the GSV was variable with almost no movement observed in some instances and large amounts in others. The difference in flow was primarily due to the change in the diameter of the vein rather than the velocity of the blood moving up the leg. This variation of flow during exercise has been demonstrated in other studies from our laboratory. [3]

These data from this small study suggest that the propulsive force in the GSV is generated from the deep plantar venous plexus. There is of course no other obvious source of propulsion. The blood collected from the saphenous tributaries could not contribute to the flow velocity.

These findings also suggest that much of the time the saphenous is simply a local collecting vessel which directs blood to the deep system but does not actively transmit it upward.

Further study is required to understand more fully the function of the foot pump and its contribution to the return of blood to the heart.

Calf muscle pump

The calf pump is formed by the muscles contained within the anterior, lateral and posterior muscular compartments. They act in a sequential and synchronized manner during walking. Figure 2.2 illustrates the global response of blood flow to the contraction of the entire calf muscle pump.

In the initial phase the distal calf pump is activated. This is initiated by dorsiflexion of the foot as the leg is lifted to take a step. Contraction of the anterior compartment muscles dorsiflexes the foot and empties its veins i.e. the anterior tibial veins. Dorsiflexion passively tightens the Achilles tendon whose constriction empties blood from the lower portions of the peroneal and posterior tibial veins.

As the foot strikes the ground, weight bearing activates the second phase, the foot pump, which has just been described. Plantar flexion initiates the third phase as the foot comes up on its toes. Contraction of the muscles of the posterior compartments, particularly the gastrocnemius and soleus, empties the proximal venous reservoir. Plantar flexion also tenses and shortens the Achilles tendon which maintains the empty state of the distal portion of the pump.

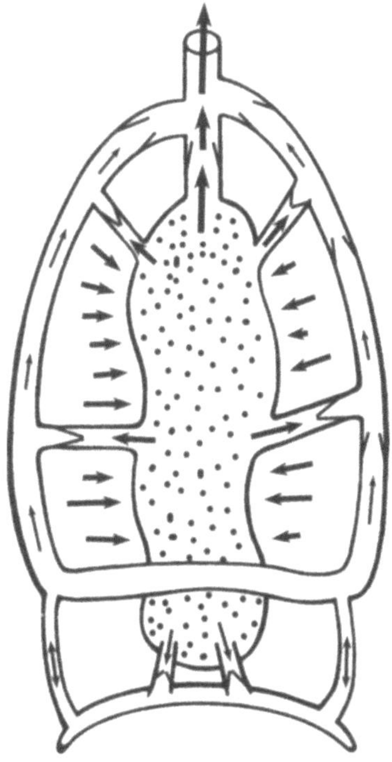

Figure 2.2 During the contraction of the calf muscles the lower valves of the tibial veins close, as do those of the saphenous perforating veins. Blood is forced out through the popliteal and femoral veins. There may be little or no flow through the saphenous veins during this phase of walking.

Other pumps

Although the foot and calf muscle pumps are the most vigorous in emptying the leg of blood other muscle groups contribute to the upward flow of blood.

Popliteal vein pump

Videophlebography shows that contraction of the gastrocnemius and popliteus muscles causes some lateral compression of the popliteal vein during plantar flexion of the ankle. [1]

Hach has also demonstrated radiographically that "when the calf muscles contract the lumen of the popliteal vein is compressed to a narrow slit by the expanding gastrocnemius muscle bellies". When relaxed the vessel immediately resumes its original caliber. [2] Repetitive muscle activities such as walking and bike riding appear to have a significant hemodynamic effect on blood velocity through the popliteal vein.

Superficial femoral vein pump

As the femoral vein enters the thigh through Hunter's canal it is compressed by the *quadriceps* and *sartorius muscles.* The increased velocity of compression is especially pronounced in professional cyclists where the sartorius becomes hypertrophied. [2] Flexion of the knee by contracting the hamstrings also incites flow in the common femoral vein. Although the deep femoral vein drains into the superficial femoral vein it collects blood mostly from the muscles of the posterior thigh and gluteal region. Few quantitative data are available from the action of these muscles.

Refilling the pump

The emptied calf veins refill from arterial inflow and from the veins of the superficial system and the foot veins. Trendelenburg in his famous 1891 epistle gave a perfect description of the arterial refilling time. [4]

When the muscles have contracted and expelled their blood there is no pressure within the deep system. On the other hand the surface veins are full of blood and subject to hydrostatic pressure. A pressure gradient of perhaps 100 mmHg exists between the two systems. Therefore after the expulsion of blood the deep veins fill immediately from the superficial veins via the many perforating veins and the saphenous junctions which connect the two systems. This response is diagrammatically represented in Fig. 2.3.

Concomitant with the emptying of the superficial and deep venous compartments is a drop of venous pressure.

Venous pressure

In large part the pressure within the veins determines their general health. Unlike the arterial system where the pressure remains relatively constant, the venous pressure varies greatly from one part of the system to another.

Intramuscular pressure

Because of the enormous pressures generated within the confines of the muscular compartments, the valvular integrity of the perforating and communicating veins is especially important for normal functioning.

The intramuscular veins, e.g. gastocnemius and soleus, may be forcibly compressed during contraction

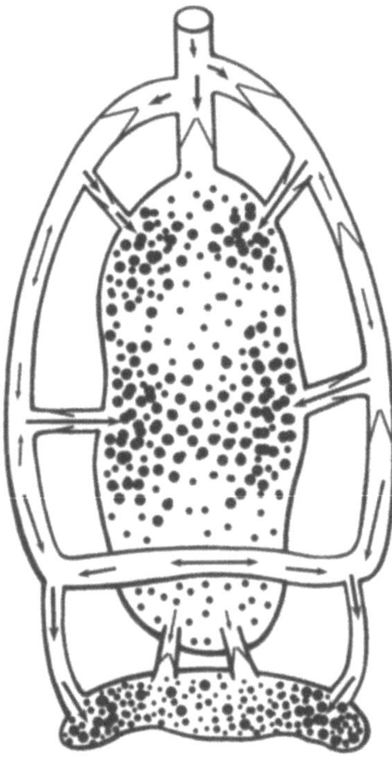

Figure 2.3 The leg is at rest and the surface veins empty quickly into the deep venous system. The foot pump is filled by its perforating veins. The saphenous systems have collected blood from the skin and subcutaneous tissues and drain into the calf and thigh veins.

by pressures of 200–300 mmHg. APG measurements show that an average 170 lb man may expel as much as 80 ml or more of blood from the calf with each step he takes. This volume may increase as ambulation proceeds due to exercise hyperemia of the muscles.

The intermuscular veins lying outside the muscles but within the compartments are also forcibly compressed. Although not compressed as directly by muscular contractions, pressures of perhaps 100–200 mmHg are reported. This group consists of the anterior and posterior tibial, and the peroneal veins, all of which have received blood from the foot and the perforating veins. [5]

From the high pressures generated in the calf and foot the blood is transferred into the popliteal and femoral veins which form a large volume, low resistance outflow tract.

Transmural pressure

Most veins assume an elliptical or dumbbell shape when empty. When filled with blood they become round. Their cross-sectional area and hence their volume may be three to four times that of a corresponding artery.

The hemodynamic characteristics of a vein depend on its *transmural pressure* which represents the pressure gradient across the vein wall. This is the difference between the intravenous pressure which distends the vein and the external forces which try to collapse it.

When a vein is incompletely filled, its intraluminal pressure remains relatively low. Nor is there a significant change in pressure as the vein fills. It is only when the vein is completely filled and distended with blood that the pressure increases. At this point a small increase of volume causes a large change in pressure. This response is shown in Fig. 2.4 wherein the vein enlarges with little change in pressure until it is filled.

Venous pressure is especially affected by position and activity. Other factors including temperature, valvular competence and cardiorespiratory function contribute to pressure changes as well. However, the pressure in veins is seldom less than 5 mmHg, below which they collapse. Pressure gradients and their alterations ultimately determine the health of the venous system.

Ambulatory venous pressure (AVP)

Normally arterial blood is pumped from the left ventricle at a pressure of at least 120 mmHg. As blood passes through the arterial system there is a gradual diminution of pressure. After blood passes the arteriolar capillary bed a pressure of about 15 mmHg is transmitted to the venous side. This residual pressure in the vein is called *vis a tergo*. When a person is lying flat, *vis a tergo* provides enough energy to return blood to the right heart, where the pressure may be only 0–3 mmHg.

When the person stands up, however, hydrostatic pressure adds a tremendous force. On the venous side of the circulation the hydrostatic pressure represents the weight of the column of blood in the veins connecting the right atrium and the foot.

Trendelenburg thought that healthy valves protected the legs from the hydrostatic pressure generated in the valveless vena cava. We now know from direct measurements that hydrostatic pressure is transmitted through the venous network from heart to foot regardless of the health of the valvular system.

When a person changes from a lying to a standing position arteriolar blood slowly fills the veins. According to the volume and pressure relationship outlined above, the pressure increases gradually with the filling of the veins. Depending on the height of the person the ultimate standing pressure may reach 100 mmHg in a superficial foot vein. This pressure represents the weight of the column of blood between the right heart and the foot. Therefore the static standing pressure is the same whether the venous system is normal or whether it is totally abnormal.

However, during exercise the muscular activity of the calf and foot expels blood from the leg. According to the same volume/pressure relationship, emptying the venous bed reduces the venous pressure.

A healthy leg muscle pump can reduce the pressure in the foot by 60–80%, from 100 to 20 mmHg within a number of seconds. The minimum pressure obtained during exercise is called the *ambulatory venous pressure* (AVP).

With cessation of exercise it normally requires 20–30 s for the pressure in the emptied veins to return to pre-exercise levels, e.g. 100 mmHg. This pressure change coincides with the refilling of the venous bed from arterial inflow. This phase of the cycle is called the venous refilling time (VRT or just RT).

When valvular incompetence is present the venous reservoir is filled not only from arteriolar inflow but also from blood refluxing during the resting phase between muscular contractions. In this situation the venous reservoir is never quite emptied by muscular activity and the pressure may never be reduced to the minimum level. With continued reflux the AVP remains elevated during exercise.

The refilling time under these circumstances is usually decreased as well. That is, at the cessation of exercise the venous reservoir is only partially emptied from the previous contraction and the time required to refill it is thereby reduced. Reflux continues from the current contraction and provides extra blood to refill it even more quickly. In the disease state the RT may decrease to 10 s or less. Figure 2.5 shows a printout of a normal AVP test. When abnormal the pressure tracing does not decrease and the RT is more rapid with a steep uphill slant.

It is of interest to note that Trendelenburg described the refilling time in his famous work of 1891. After

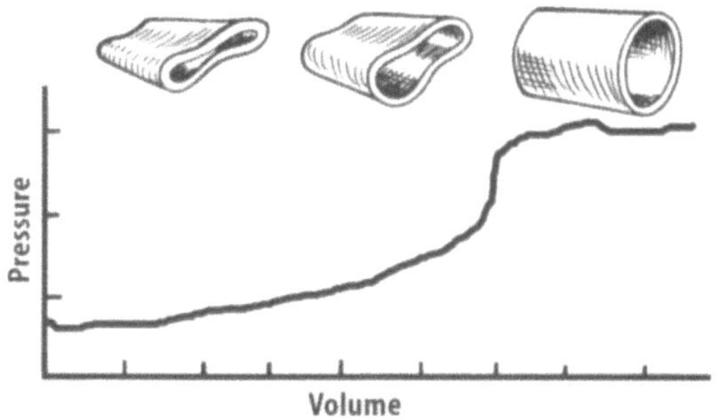

Figure 2.4 This simplified diagram shows the relationship between volume and pressure. As long as the vein is incompletely filled and flaccid there is little change in pressure. When the vein becomes distended there is a sudden and marked increase in the intraluminal pressure.

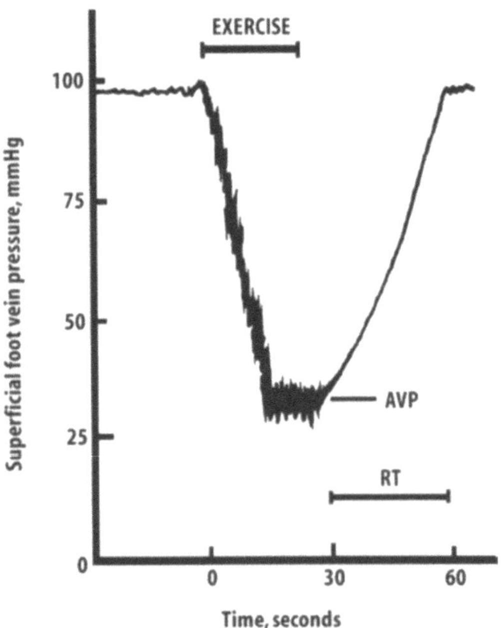

Figure 2.5 This drawing demonstrates the normal changes in pressure measured in a superficial vein on the dorsum of the foot. When the subject is standing quietly the pressure is around 100 mmHg, which represents the hydrostatic pressure measured from the heart to the foot. As the patient exercises the pressure gradually decreases until a steady state is obtained. This pressure level is the ambulatory venous pressure (AVP). Once exercise is stopped the veins refill from arteriolar inflow. The refilling time (RT) is about 25–30 s during which the resting pressure returns to former levels.

emptying the leg by elevation, compressing the saphenous junction and standing the patient he observed, "We see that the whole saphenous vein now remains empty at first on standing. Not until the lapse of a quarter to a half a minute does one see the varicosities in the leg gradually begin to fill with blood again."

Central venous pressure (CVP)

Central venous pressure is the pressure in the central portion of the venous system. It represents the combined forces of blood returning to the heart. CVP is usually measured in the superior vena cava or right atrium.

The measurement of CVP is fairly simple. A central catheter line is placed and attached to a water manometer. The venous pressure is read directly from the level of water in the manometer. In the normal individual it measures 3–10 cm H_2O, and remains fairly constant even with changes in position.

CVP is often monitored by surgeons to help determine the amount of blood loss during surgery.

It is also useful in determining the degree of hydration in a patient. There is little relationship between CVP and venous diseases of the legs.

An elevation of CVP, as found in heart failure, can increase the venous pressure in the legs with secondary edema. These changes are reversible with treatment of the cardiac failure. Little permanent damage is found when the cause of the disease process is identified and treated.

Chronic venous insufficiency (CVI)

The state of persistently elevated AVP, described above, is called *chronic venous hypertension*. The causes of venous insufficiency and venous hypertension are examined below.

Classification of CVI

Two classifications of CVI are generally recognized in the USA. The first was prepared in 1988 by a subcommittee of the Society for Vascular Surgery and the International Society for Cardiovascular Surgery. [6] The committee describes CVI as "an abnormally functioning venous system caused by venous valvular incompetence with or without associated venous outflow obstruction, which may affect the superficial venous system, the deep venous system or both. The venous dysfunction may result from congenital or acquired processes."

1988 classification

This classification system is based on the severity of clinical signs and symptoms and the degree of cutaneous changes.

- Class 0: asymptomatic. Here there are some signs of chronic venous disease, varicose veins, early skin changes or other evidence of venous incompetence but without physical symptoms or alteration in function.

- Class 1: mild CVI with signs and symptoms including mild to moderate ankle swelling, mild discomfort (e.g. sensation of leg heaviness or painful varicosities), and local or generalized dilatation of subcutaneous veins. In this clinical class, CVI is usually limited to involvement of the superficial veins only.

- Class 2: moderate CVI including hyperpigmentation of the skin in the gaiter area, moderate brawny edema, and subcutaneous fibrosis, which may be either limited in extent or involve the entire malleolar and pretibial area but without ulceration. There is usually prominent local and regional dilatation of the subcutaneous veins, i.e. varicose veins.
- Class 3: severe CVI. Chronic distal leg pain associated with ulceration or pre-ulcerative skin changes, eczematoid changes, and/or severe edema. This category is usually associated with extensive involvement of the deep venous system with widespread loss of venous valvular function and/or chronic deep vein obstruction.

This system is simple and has contributed to a better understanding of diagnosis and treatment results. However, the rapid expansion of knowledge of chronic venous disease has demanded a more precise method of classification.

1994 classification

To correct this deficiency a new classification was developed at a consensus meeting of phlebologists in Maui Hawaii, February 1994. [7] It provides a more uniform and precise basis for assessing and reporting various modalities of diagnosis and treatment. The classification utilizes the following headings:

C is for clinical signs (grade 0–6) supplemented by (A) for asymptomatic and (S) for symptomatic presentation.

The clinical classifications are:

- Class 0: no visible or palpable signs of venous disease
- Class 1: telangiectasias or reticular veins
- Class 2: varicose veins
- Class 3: edema
- Class 4: skin changes ascribed to venous disease (e.g. pigmentation, venous eczema, lipodermatosclerosis)
- Class 5: skin changes as defined above with healed ulceration
- Class 6: skin changes as defined above with active ulceration

Thus a patient with primary varicose veins which cause aching or pain would be assigned the classification of (C2,S).

E is for etiologic classification (congenital, primary, secondary). The designation would then be (EC), (EP)

with undetermined cause or (ES) with known cause, e.g. post-thrombotic, post-traumatic or other recognizable cause. A is for anatomic distribution (superficial, deep, or perforator, alone or in combination). For reports requiring greater detail the site and extent of involvement can be included from a list of anatomic segments. P is for pathophysiologic dysfunction (reflux or obstruction alone or in combination). More precise descriptions can also be included from the anatomic segments use in the anatomic category.

Because this classification is relatively new it is undergoing evaluation and will probably need revision. In the mean time it provides a more definitive method of reporting.

Compensated CVI

I like to think of CVI as being compensated or uncompensated. My definition of compensated CVI includes all cases of major venous diseases without major complication. It includes superficial saphenous incompetence with varicose veins. It also includes a leg with varicosis from previous DVT but with no other complications. It might include non-saphenous varicosis as well. Many of these patients will have minor symptoms but no other complication.

For example one sees many patients with huge varicosis of many years' duration with marked reflux in the saphenous trunks but with only minor symptoms, little functional alteration and no skin changes. In general this leg has been able to compensate for the reflux, although the saphenous tributaries have become varicose. The muscle pumps have apparently been able to overcome the overload of blood resulting from the reflux. In this group the AVP remains in a range that is sufficiently normal for no complications to develop.

Uncompensated CVI

In this category the symptoms are more severe and skin changes are obvious. The muscle pump can no longer keep up with the task of emptying the venous reservoir and the AVP remains elevated. This condition is more likely where there is deep vein incompetence but is not at all uncommon in patients who have pure superficial incompetence.

As the venous system continues to decompensate and venous pressure cannot be controlled the condition is termed "chronic venous hypertension".

Chronic venous hypertension (CVH)

In the broadest hemodynamic sense, venous hypertension develops when exercise can no longer empty the leg of blood and decrease the ambulatory venous pressure to normal levels. Recall that venous volume can increase in the unfilled vein with little or no increase in pressure. However, the pressure in the filled venous reservoir increases rapidly with an increase of volume. Many centers have verified that the chronic, non-embolic complications of venous disease, e.g. liposclerosis and ulcers, are almost universally associated with an elevated ambulatory venous pressure and persistent venous hypertension.

Etiology of CVI and CVH

Of the various causes for venous insufficiency, compensated and uncompensated, two major causative factors are apparent: calf pump failure and venous reflux from valvular incompetence.

Primary pump failure

Many non-venous conditions can prevent the pumps from functioning properly. Paralysis, muscle weakness, immobilization by long car rides or by casts prevent foot and calf pumps from performing their usual function.

Venous diseases themselves may contribute to pumping failure. Liposclerosis, ulceration and lymphedema often immobilize the ankle. In these conditions the calf muscles may be normal but cannot contract during ambulation with subsequent loss of pumping action.

The calf muscles and their valvular system may also be damaged by injury, infection or DVT with subsequent inadequate function.

Valvular incompetence with reflux

Reflux, the retrograde flow of blood, occurs when valvular competence is lost and is the common denominator of chronic venous disease. Most phlebologists classify the loss of competence as primary or secondary.

Primary valvular incompetence

This condition is defined wherein the venous system itself is normal but where valvular function has been compromised, usually from stretching of the vein wall. Several congenital vascular diseases are associated with valvular incompetence and reflux. The Klippel–Trenaunay syndrome is characterized by vestigial marginal veins and undeveloped or absent deep veins. Valvular agenesis is described with incompetent saphenous trunks and varicose surface veins. This syndrome is illustrated in Figures 3.1 and 4.9.

Men with varicose veins and no intervening venous disease may have primary valvular or vein wall disorder. There are also some young women with varicose veins and no pregnancy who fall into this category. The problem is usually one of saphenous vein incompetence with truncal varicosities. However, idiopathic refluxes of the deep venous system associated with superficial varicosis are well documented.

When examined by a variety of means, one usually finds a dilated vein with incompetent but otherwise healthy valves. The pathogenesis of this situation develops into the chicken and egg controversy. One side argues a genetically inadequate valvular structure. It malfunctions and reflux develops. Dilation of the vein follows the reflux. The other side contests that the vein wall is congenitally weak, cannot tolerate normal venous pressure and dilates. Dilation distracts the valve cusps and reflux occurs. While this entire area of speculation is open to further research, current thinking tends to favor the latter faulty-wall theory. [8]

Figure 2.6 illustrates the overflow of blood from the femoral vein into an incompetent saphenous vein. When the pumps are at rest the refluxing blood enters the deep systems. Continued reflux engorges the venous reservoir. There may be no evidence of venous hypertension if the muscular pumps can continue to empty the leg of blood in spite of the continued overload. If, however, the pumps cannot compensate for the overload, venous hypertension develops and the signs of venous insufficiency emerge.

Recirculation

Trendelenburg first outlined the concept that the recirculation of refluxing blood created an *independent* circulation of its own. Perthes attributes Trendelenburg as calling it a "privater Kreislauf", i.e. *private circulation*. [9] Hach recently furthered the idea by calling it "Die Rezirkulationkreise", the *recirculation circle*. [10]

Our exercise testing confirms the idea that active retrograde flow occurs down an incompetent saphenous during exercise and is only interrupted by the contraction of the calf muscles. Many laboratories

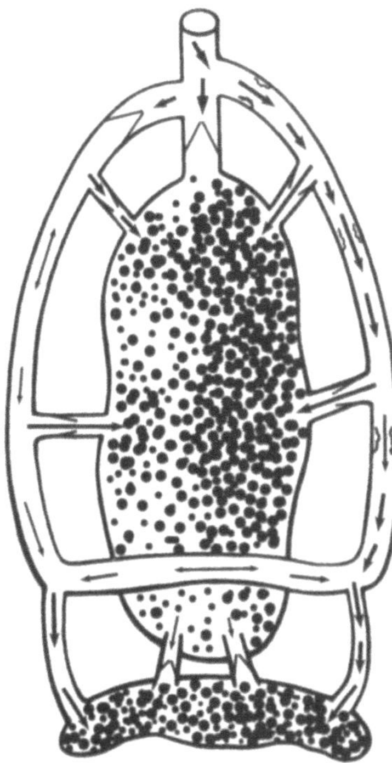

Figure 2.6 Incompetent valves are shown along the greater saphenous vein. During exercise blood refluxes from the femoral vein to re-enter the thigh, calf and foot veins. The efficiency of these muscle pumps may decrease because of the overload from the refluxing blood. As long as the pumps can evacuate the excess blood volume and maintain a normal ambulatory venous pressure the leg remains relatively normal. If the pumps fail to relieve the pressure then the complications of venous hypertension develop.

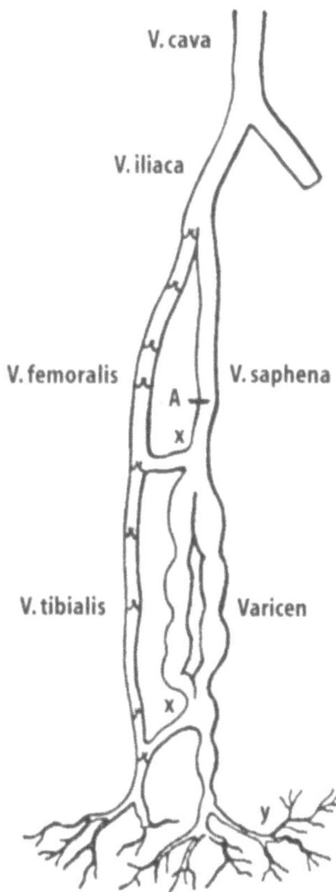

Figure 2.7 Trendelenburg's understanding of venous flow is beautifully illustrated in this drawing. He shows a normally valved deep venous system but no valvular function in the iliac and greater saphenous system. Each "*x*" marks the perforating veins which return the overflowing blood to the deep veins. The "varicen" (varicosities) are the huge bubbly veins of advanced disease. The "*y*" is the network of filling capillaries and venules. "*A*" marks the spot where he performed ligation and division of the saphenous vein, usually in the low thigh where the vein began to bulge.

have also confirmed an improvement of deep venous function after treating superficial disease.

Figure 2.7 is from Trendelenburg's paper and shows the diseased and valveless saphenous vein. He says that, "…as soon as the muscles begin to work the pumping action of the venous valves in the deep system come into play. As a result the blood stream in the deep veins will move appreciably faster and the blood will be sucked through the communicating veins, "*x*".

He described the resulting blood flow. "It will not remain away because the blood from the reservoir of the filled saphenous flows after it and is replaced from the femoral vein above, so that in this case we are dealing with an *independent circulation* of the lower leg, so to say, in that the blood of the leg's deep veins is pumped up and partly flows down again through the saphenous."

Pregnancy

Probably the largest group of patients in the category of primary insufficiency are women who have had children. They have perfectly normal veins until they become pregnant. But the hormonal stimulation coupled with intra-abdominal pressure and increased blood volume dilates the venous systems rendering the valves incompetent. Continued local venous hypertension dilates the saphenous tributaries causing them to become varicose.

During pregnancy estrogen and progesterone levels are escalating, especially during the first trimester. Many women know that they are pregnant because their veins suddenly become painful. The relaxing effects of the hormones on the venous system begin as early as this. An increased blood volume fills and stretches the relaxed veins of the legs. Add an enlarging uterus to impede venous return and you get a mother with varicose veins. Many women are fortunate that their veins shrink after delivery and many of the varicose veins return to normal. However, many women are left with residual varicosities. Fortunately this problem is reasonably easy to treat.

Secondary valvular incompetence

In this situation the loss of valvular function in a previously normal venous system is associated with a specific disease process, usually DVT. A basic question to be answered when evaluating the causes of reflux is whether there is or has been outflow obstruction.

Deep venous outflow obstruction

The most common cause of deep venous obstruction is deep venous thrombosis (DVT). The effects of obstruction may be either temporary or permanent. Generally, the more proximal the obstruction in the venous system the greater the venous insufficiency. It is obvious that DVT of the iliofemoral tract blocks much more flow than a DVT in the calf muscles.

A thrombosis in the calf veins may develop few obstructive problems. Blood from the foot and ankle is easily diverted into the superficial veins with little alteration in valvular function. Of course DVT in the calf muscles may alter the pumping capability of the muscles with subsequent incomplete emptying and back-up of blood. DVT in the major drainage veins, popliteal, femoral and iliac, however, usually causes major backflow problems, at least temporarily. Blockage of the these principal outflow pathways creates a progressive back-up of blood within the venous reservoir. When the reservoir can no longer compensate for the increasing volume, venous hypertension ensues. The ability of the calf pump to empty the leg and reduce ambulatory venous pressure determines the long-term effects of blockage.

The size and extent of DVT is also important in determining the ultimate degree of venous insufficiency. A small DVT of the femoral vein, for example, may recanalize quickly. The obstructive effects, dilation of the distal venous system by reflux, may be reversed as the obstruction disappears and little permanent damage is done.

Usually there are more permanent sequelae of DVT. For example the DVT may not recanalize and forms a permanent fibrous scar which blocks or distorts the vein. Continued venous distention renders otherwise normal valves incompetent and the ensuing reflux allows further dilation of the venous reservoir. If the calf muscle pump fails to empty the ever-increasing blood volume venous hypertension becomes entrenched and the secondary complications develop.

One of the more prominent side-effects of obstruction is the development of collateral vessels as the obstructed blood finds other channels to the heart. There are many natural collaterals in the deep system which can bypass the obstructed vein. For example drainage from the foot can pass directly into the superficial system when necessary and obstructed calf veins can divert their blood among the adjacent veins.

In the thigh the deep femoral system can divert blood via pudendal and gluteal veins into the internal iliac and gonadal veins. The superficial system becomes a collateral only when the perforating veins become incompetent. Competent valves within the system of perforating veins ordinarily protect the superficial system from the high pressures generated within the calf muscle pump. When the outflow of the pump is obstructed the force is directed into the perforating veins. If their walls expand from continued high pressure their valves become incompetent. The venous hypertension of the deep veins is then transmitted directly into the superficial system.

Pelvic tumors

Pelvic masses or tumors would seem to be an obvious cause of altered venous return. Unless the tumor invades the pelvic veins directly there is seldom significant obstruction to venous flow. An otherwise healthy calf pump can overcome the slight increase in resistance and maintain a healthy leg.

Inferior vena caval interruption

During the 1960s it was common practice in the USA to surgically clip or tie off the inferior vena cava to prevent pulmonary embolization following DVT. Those patients who have been able to develop adequate intra-abdominal collaterals have had few problems. However, many patients have developed marked venous insufficiency of the legs with concomitant complications such as chronic swelling, lymphedema and ulceration. The obstructive process is a cause of "venous claudication". The patient cannot walk more than 10–20 yards before the engorged legs cause pain. The patient whose huge ulcer is shown in Fig. 9.3 was handicapped in this way.

Other organic disease can cause venous insufficiency. Congestive heart failure is a well-known cause of acute venous insufficiency. The word "congestive" implies that the venous system is congested with extra blood which the heart cannot pump away. The lungs fill with blood and fluid exudes from the capillaries, the liver enlarges as it becomes congested and finally the legs become swollen. This condition is reversible when the heart is treated.

Secondary varicose veins

An important factor in the development of venous insufficiency is the extent of venous damage created by the DVT. Usually there is direct injury to the adjacent vein walls and valves. If the damage is not completely healed the damaged valves permit reflux to extend to the distal parts of the system.

DVT may also injure the perforating veins directly, permitting reflux from the deep into the superficial system. This reflux coupled with direct saphenous reflux causes many tributaries to become varicose.

Thus the long-term hemodynamic effects of DVT depend on the degree and duration of obstruction, the area of obstruction, the amount of direct damage to adjacent veins and valves, and the effect on adjacent muscle pumps.

Complications of CVH

These complications of CVI and CVH encompass a distinctive series of anatomic changes in the lower leg. Traditionally the changes were thought to be late sequelae of DVT. The terms commonly used to describe these conditions were the "post-phlebitic leg", the "post-thrombotic syndrome" and "stasis ulcer". [11]

The features common to the development of CVI are continued reflux unresponsive to muscle pump activity, engorgement of the venous reservoir and the development of chronic venous hypertension. The anatomic alterations, usually in the skin and subcutaneous tissues, may take many years to develop. As the pump fails to reduce ambulatory venous pressure, hypertension in larger veins is sequentially transmitted to the smaller collecting veins. Once-healthy veins become dilated by the elevated intraluminal pressure, their valves rendered incompetent and the hypertension is transmitted to the next set of smaller veins or venules. The final insult is to the microcirculation of the skin and subcutaneous fat.

The following complications and their treatments are described and illustrated more completely in Chaps 3 and 9:

- white atrophy
- eczematoid dermatitis
- neurodermatitis
- edema

- ulceration
- lipodermatosclerosis

Comments

While the advances in ultrasound technology and other non-invasive testing techniques give us a better understanding of normal venous anatomy and function they also increase the demand to understand the abnormal changes of form and function. Fortunately our investigations are progressing from the traditional anatomic to the histo-chemico-immunologic. Continued research may very well elucidate the causative factors and pathologic changes found with CVI so that we can better treat or perhaps prevent these complications.

References

1. Gardner AMN, Fox RH (1993) The Return of Blood to the Heart, 2nd rev ed. John Libbey, London
2. Hach W, Hach-Wunderle V (1997) Phlebography and sonography of the veins. Springer, Heidelberg
3. Tretbar LL (1995) Hemodynamic alterations in the greater saphenous vein before and after externally banded valvuloplasty. In Phlebology '95, Negus D et al eds, Phlebology, Suppl 1:370–372
4. Trendelenburg F (1891) Ueber die Unterbindung der Vena Saphena Magna Unterschenkelvaricen. Beitr zur Klin Chir, Sieb Band. Laupp'schen, Tübingen
5. Brouse NL, Burnand KG, Lea Thomas M (1988) Diseases of the veins, pathology, diagnosis and treatment. Edward Arnold, London
6. Porter JM, Rutherford RB, Clagett GP, Cranley JJ et al (1988) Reporting standards in venous disease. J Vasc Surg 8:172–181
7. Venous Consensus Conference (Feb 1994) Maui, Hawaii
8. Rose SS (1986) Some thoughts of the aetiology of varicose veins. J Cardiovasc Surg 27:534–543
9. Perthes G (1895) Ueber die operation der unterschenkelvaricen nach Trendelenburg. Deutsche Medicin Wochenschr 16:253–257
10. Hach W, Hach-Wunderle V (1994) Die Rezirkulationkreise der Primaren Varicose. Springer-Verlag, Berlin
11. Homans J (1917) The etiology and treatment of varicose ulcer of the leg. Surg Gynecol Obstet 24:300–311

CHAPTER 3

Clinical Phlebologic Evaluation

When a patient presents to the doctor's office it is tempting to ignore the complaints and initiate a series of technologic investigations. However, a carefully taken history and physical examination are as important in the field of phlebology as in other medical areas. The findings will help one to understand the nature of the venous problem and to formulate a plan for further investigation and treatment.

History of present illness

Because many venous diseases are slowly progressive and often silent in their development, current complaints may become apparent many years after the etiologic event. A thorough historical review is therefore essential. Many small changes go unnoticed or are coincidental with events of more serious consequence so that they seem trifling in proportion. The patient should be questioned about the following problems.

Onset and progression

The early changes of many primary venous diseases such as reticular varicosities and telangiectasias are noticed during teenage and early adult years. Particular attention is paid to events which may indicate a previous phlebitis or DVT. Post-partum DVT, once called "milk leg" or "white leg", is one of those events. It was so-called because the thrombosis in the deep veins started when the milk "came in" after delivery. It is relatively uncommon today because of better prenatal care, weight control

and early ambulation. Nevertheless its occurrence should be diagnosed, especially in the older age group.

Other factors commonly associated with DVT should be identified, e.g. prolonged immobilization, bed rest, trauma or surgery. When no other causative factors are apparent many people find a positive family history for varicose veins. The significance of hereditary factors remains to be clarified.

Symptoms

Curiously there is often little or no relationship between the degree of venous disease and the manifestation of symptoms. Huge clusters of varicosities may have no symptoms whereas some of the smallest clusters of spider veins may sting and burn. When present, symptoms may be specific or general in nature and are usually relegated to the lower leg.

Actual pain is sometimes reported. More often the symptoms are of a lesser degree: throbbing, aching, stinging and burning are common complaints.

Intense itching is a common complaint. The whole leg may itch or, as is often the case, the pruritic area is restricted to the skin overlying large varicose veins. Constant scratching causes a neurodermatitis for which the patient may have already been treated, the underlying venous disorder having been overlooked.

Complaints referable to position and activity are important. Pooling of blood from immobility or from standing and sitting often causes symptoms. Exercise will sometimes relieve complaints if the calf pump can empty the pooled blood and decrease ambulatory pressure. The converse may also be true. Exercise may aggravate the symptoms when the pooled blood cannot be emptied.

The worst pain is that from "venous claudication". In this situation calf pain is precipitated by walking and not particularly relieved by rest. Here there is obstruction to the outflow of blood from the leg, usually as a result of an old DVT. Exercise creates hyperemia of the leg and pain develops when the muscle pumps cannot evacuate the extra blood. Arterial claudication is differentiated by the disappearance of pain by rest and the ability to walk on after resting.

Sometimes venous symptoms are nocturnal. Cramps or muscle pain will awaken the patient. Because he may get relief from walking (as does the patient with arterial insufficiency) it is necessary to differentiate the two causative factors.

Pregnancy

Many varicose veins begin during pregnancy. They may recede following the birth only to enlarge after the next pregnancy. The patient may also recall the presence of vulval or pudendal varices during pregnancy but may not associate them with the current venous problem.

Effect of menstrual cycle

Many women complain of symptoms just before or at the beginning of their period. Many veins, both large and small, are sensitized by the elevated hormone levels late in the menstrual cycle. The veins become tender to touch and sting and burn. Pudendal and vulval veins are particularly sensitive to these changes.

Other symptoms of the "premenstrual syndrome" should be investigated. Fluid retention may be a prominent feature with some of the fluid deposited in the dilated and sensitized veins. When other parts of the body become sensitive and swollen the same reaction occurs in the veins.

Vulvopudendal varices

Patients with these varices may also experience marked pelvic symptoms during the premenstrual period. This complex has been called the "pelvic congestion syndrome". It is the result of extensive pelvic varices developing during pregnancy. Apparently the pelvic varices are sensitized by the hormonal changes and expand with fluid. Pelvic heaviness, dyspareunia, dysuria, and painful bowel movements are reported.

Vulvopudendal varices are an extension of the pelvic varices. Figure 5.7 illustrates this varicose problem. Venous hypertension begins in the pelvic and ovarian veins and is transmitted to the thigh and lower leg. The women may not associate the pelvic and leg symptoms until asked about them.

Effect of previous treatment

The response to prior treatment may give a clue to the factors responsible for the development of new varicosities. Early recurrence, e.g. within a year or so, suggests incomplete or inappropriate treatments or an inaccurate diagnosis. Slowly developing symptoms or disease suggests the natural progression of the disease.

Bad circulation

Many people complain about "bad circulation". Often they are referring to cold, blue, or purple feet. These complaints usually are irrelevant to the venous evaluation. However, such complaints should not be taken lightly because they may represent genuine symptoms of arterial disease. The response to cold is also important. The painful, blue toes (and fingers) of Raynaud's phenomenon may be the actual problem which the patient believes is venous in origin.

Past medical history

Congestive heart failure

Heart failure is usually accompanied with an increased blood volume. The failing heart cannot empty the venous bed and the "congestion" causes peripheral edema. One must watch for a sudden exacerbation of distal venous problems, e.g. ulceration, as a result of heart failure.

Renal and pulmonary failure

These processes may also exacerbate peripheral venous disease. Healed venous ulcers have been known to break open during a period of renal failure. An otherwise asymptomatic DVT may activate pulmonary failure with showers of pulmonary emboli.

Arterial vascular disease

As noted previously, venous and arterial disease can exhibit similar symptoms. Cutaneous ulcerations much like those of venous origin may be seen with the small vessel disease found in diabetes or rheumatoid arthritis.

Autoimmune diseases

Patients with rheumatoid diseases can develop severe leg ulcers mimicking venous ulcers. Hypercoagulable states are associated with some immune diseases such as lupus.

Familial hypercoagulability

Although this is not a common problem, a history of unexpected and recurrent DVTs can be elicited in some families. Appropriate testing is necessary to evaluate this congenital defect. After evaluation treatment may still be appropriate for secondary conditions.

Exaggerated histamine responses

Dermatographia, spontaneous "nervous" hives, histamine flushes and histamine headaches are examples of this condition. Sclerotherapy may stimulate some of these reactions but has not been reported as a problem. Simple antihistamines will often block these unpleasant side-effects.

Allergic history

If a patient is to receive injection sclerotherapy his allergy history is important. Most of the sclerosing solutions cause a non-specific local allergic reaction when injected. However, some solutions contain specific allergenic substances. The patient should be asked about the following:

Chromium

One European sclerosant contains a chromated glycerin and may react to those with an allergy to chromium. These people usually are identified by their inability to wear chromium-containing silver-alloy jewelry.

Iodine

Iodinated compounds are also widely used as sclerosants. Some people may have had an iodine reaction to other medication or an allergic response to certain shell fish.

Bee stings

People with no prior allergic history may exhibit severe anaphylactoid reactions to various stimuli. Anecdotal stories of fatal reactions to bee stings are common. Similar non-specific reactions to injected sclerosants have also been reported. A few of these potential victims can be identified by their progressively severe reactions to insect bites.

Asthma and other allergic diseases

These patients should be carefully screened and treated to avoid exacerbation of their disease.

Local anesthetics

Many venous problems require surgical intervention under local anesthesia. Dental treatments will give the patient evidence of any reactions to local anesthesia. When an "allergic" reaction is reported from dental anesthetics one must be careful to identify whether it was a true allergic reaction or whether it was an adrenaline response associated with cardiac symptoms.

Physical examination

The patient should be undressed from the waist down. Modesty is maintained with loose-fitting shorts which allow easy access to the groin, inner thigh and pubic area. A well-lighted room is essential with a comfortable ambient temperature maintained for the partially clothed patient.

Initially the patient is examined in the standing position. It is best to have her stand on a stool or pedestal. A common stepping stool is generally not high enough. The stand should provide a hand grip for support and a surface large enough for easy turning during the examination. This type of stool is shown in Fig. 3.1.

Most people are not accustomed to being examined

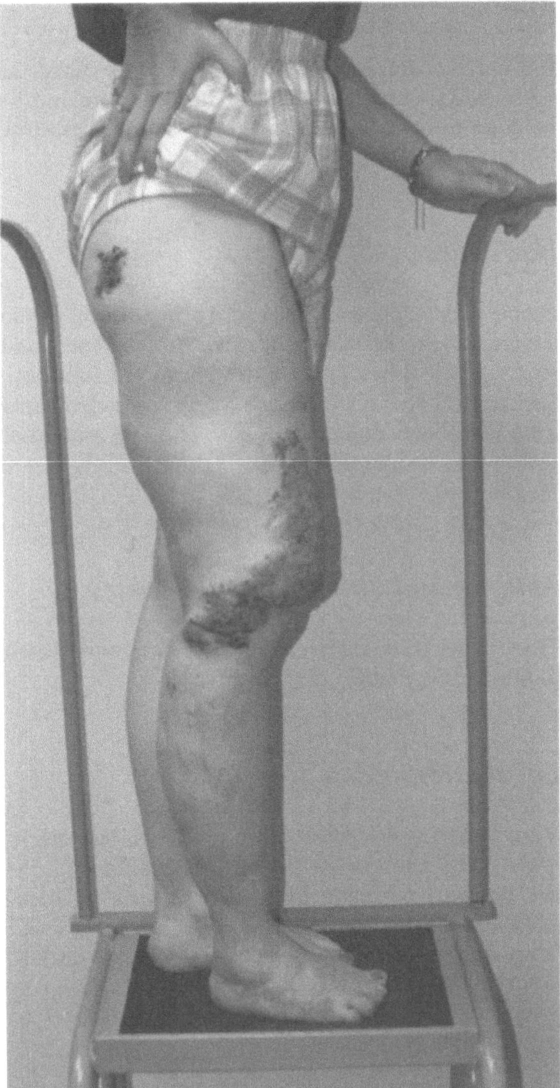

while standing, especially while elevated above the floor. They frequently become light-headed or dizzy with the static of a Doppler in the background. Watch for signs of an impending faint such as sighing, murmuring, slouching, or quietness.

Dermatologic changes

The skin, especially of the lower calf and ankle, should be inspected, tapped, touched, pressed and squeezed. It should be evaluated for temperature, texture, color, turgor, moisture and hair quality and compared to the other leg.

Pigmentation

A typical sign of CVI is the deposition of pigment, usually hemosiderin, in the skin of the lower leg and ankle. It may be absent in the foot. Figures 9.1 and 9.2 show these changes clearly. Multiple tiny red petechiae can be seen in the skin prior to the appearance of the pigment itself.

The distribution of pigment is erratic; it may be distributed circumferentially on the skin surface or may be present only on the medial ankle. It sometimes appears over large bulging varicosities as they travel up the leg but may be absent around smaller varices on the foot.

Although pigmentation has been thought to represent deep venous insufficiency, it is commonly found in superficial insufficiency as well. When caused by superficial insufficiency, it may be more localized along the course of the saphenous veins.

Pigmentation is also found over the entire calf of legs which have been treated with many kinds of salves and lotions. This allergic response is called "pigmentation medicamentosa" and may be melanin deposits rather than hemosiderin.

Lipodermatosclerosis

Also called more simply liposclerosis, this term was coined by Brouse and Bernand to describe the advanced dermatologic changes in the skin and subcutaneous fat. The term implies the sclerosis or thickening of the skin and fat found in the lower leg and ankle.

As liposclerosis progresses the skin and subcutaneous fat becomes thickened and hard, causing the area to contract. These changes are discussed more fully in Chap. 2 and depicted in Fig. 3.2.

White atrophy

Called "atrophie blanche" in French, this describes the appearance of a scar in an area of CVI. The scar is pale white due to the paucity of capillaries or pigment in the epithelium. A few tiny, pink vascular islands may punctuate the epithelium, giving it a pebbly surface. The scar is thin, fragile and poorly supported by dermis, rendering it vulnerable to minor trauma.

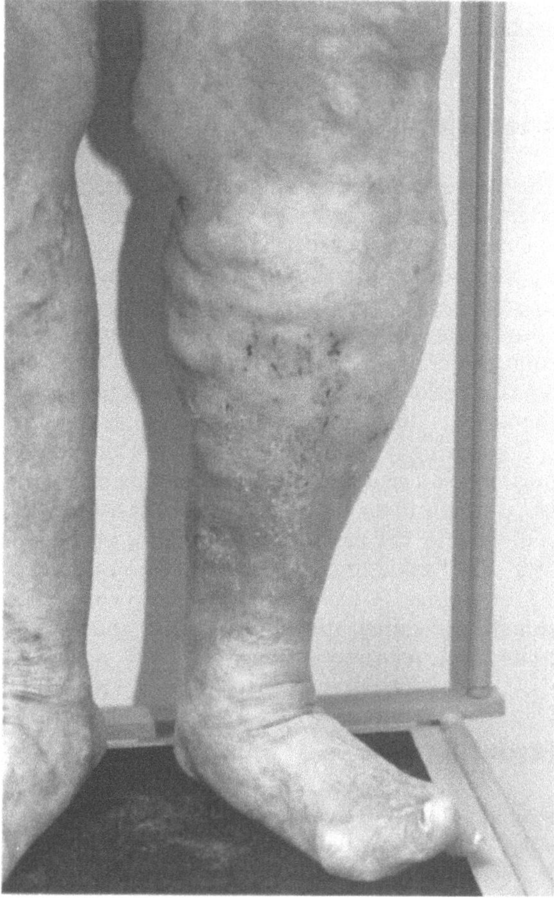

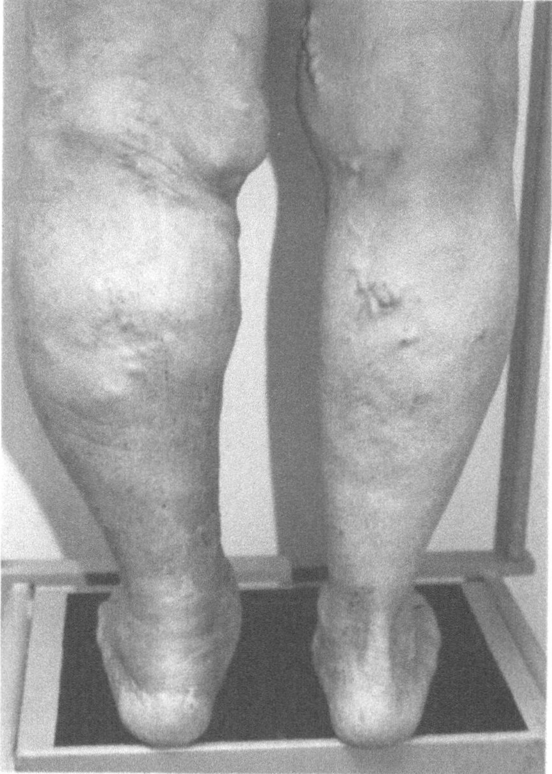

Figure 3.3 This is the same patient shown in Fig. 3.2 and demonstrates that the edema is only seen from behind. The right leg has varicose veins and some edema but is less involved than the left. Even with the narrowing from the severe liposclerotic changes the edema obscures the Achilles tendon.

Figure 3.2 The photograph shows the results of 25 years of untreated chronic venous insufficiency due to pure superficial disease. The skin of the lower leg is thickened, indurated, darkened and shrunken. The skin was intensely pruritic and scratch marks can be seen. Treatment had been denied to the patient as the changes were thought to be "post-thrombotic" in nature. The bulging greater saphenous vein at and below the knee is obvious.

On occasion the atrophic condition develops in an ischemic area of liposclerosis without previous ulceration and may herald the imminent breakdown of the skin. More often it represents the scar of a healed venous ulcer. Refer to color Plate 1 which depicts this change.

Edema

Swelling of the leg or foot is usually obvious to the examiner. However, all legs should be observed with the patient facing away. Subtle or localized swelling in some cases may only be seen from behind, next to the Achilles tendon as shown in Fig. 3.3. Measurements of the two legs at calf and ankle should be recorded. It should be noted whether the swelling is soft or hard,

whether the skin pits and whether it is painful to pressure. When venous insufficiency has been present for a long time the edema may advance to lymphedema, which is quite hard and difficult to pit. It usually involves the dorsum of the foot whereas simple venous edema involves the ankle and lower calf.

Corona phlebectatica

The "phlebectatic crown" or ankle flare is another early sign of insufficiency. Early in the process it is represented by a grouping of prominent, dilated and often reddened veins at the level of the malleoli. As the insufficiency becomes more advanced the tiny veins continue to dilate and thin out and assume a pebbly blue appearance. We call these "blue blebs". As they thin out they become fragile and bleed easily from minor trauma. The patient shown in Fig. 3.4 had diffuse saphenous vein disease associated with the corona.

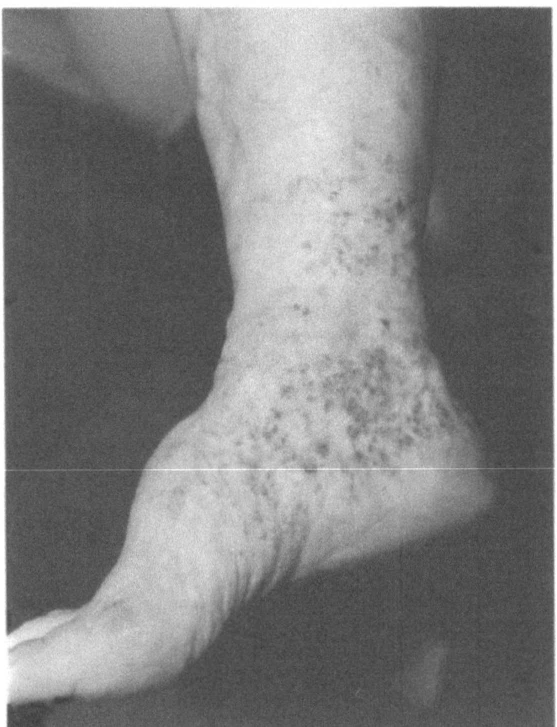

Figure 3.4 A typical ankle flare is seen here; the "blue blebs" were part of a diffuse saphenous vein disease. The patient presented at the Emergency Department with bleeding from the veins. Three episodes of bleeding had occurred during the previous year. No further bleeding occurred during the 7 years following treatment of her varicose vein disease.

Varicose veins

One should determine whether the dilated veins are branches of the two saphenous systems, that is, truncal varicosities, or varicose reticular veins. Varicose reticular veins can reach diameters of 1 cm or more but are usually quite blue in color and closer to the skin surface. When the dilated veins are reticular further testing is not usually indicated.

The position of varicose veins will usually suggest to which saphenous system they belong. Varicosities of the thigh or medial calf usually originate from the greater saphenous vein whereas those on the posterior or lateral calf usually derive from the lesser saphenous vein. Veins on the medial aspect of the knee can come from either system.

When dilated from prolonged reflux the GSV may be visible or palpable but seldom is it actually varicose. Even when grossly dilated it runs in a straight, or perhaps undulating line along its usual anatomic path. The SFJ may become varicose and protrude in the groin but any large varicosity in the thigh is probably an incompetent anterior lateral or posterior medial accessory saphenous vein. Care should be taken when examining varicosities because they may be quite tender or sensitive to touch.

Arterial insufficiency

The skin should be examined for typical signs of arterial insufficiency. Pallor of the skin on elevation and dependent rubor may be typical findings but can be confused by the skin changes of venous insufficiency. Rapid capillary refilling after pressure on the under surface of the toe is a good sign of small vessel competence. Palpation of the posterior tibial and dorsalis pedis pulses are standard procedure but flow should be confirmed by Doppler examination.

Comparing the brachial and posterior tibial artery pressures is a standard method of testing for arterial blood supply in the leg. The brachial arterial pressure is divided by the pressure measured in the ankle to create the "ankle-brachial index" (ABI). An index of 0.8 or higher is considered normal. The ABI is sometimes called the ante-brachial index. This technique is reviewed in Chap. 4.

Fascial hernia

Defects in the muscular fascia of the leg can cause a bulge which is frequently mistaken for a varicose vein by the patient. Fascial hernias are usually found in mid calf over the anterior tibial muscle just lateral to the tibia. They measure 0.5–1 cm in diameter, are usually bilateral and flatter than varicoses. When the bulging skin is compressed the fascial defect is easily felt.

The *toe-up test* differentiates between hernia and varicose vein. Ask the patient to hold on to the stand and rock back on his heels. The bulge flattens as the anterior tibial muscle tightens. Doppler examination fails to identify blood in the bulge. Figure 3.5 demonstrates the results of this test.

Trendelenburg test

Although Trendelenburg's name was attached to tourniquet testing in 1891, Brodie described the method some 45 years earlier (see Chap. 6). It is therefore properly called the *Brodie–Trendelenburg test* [1,2]. The test is a method of detecting reflux from the greater or lesser saphenous veins and from perforating veins along the course of the saphenous trunks. In clinical practice it has been used to determine the source of reflux causing varicose veins in the leg.

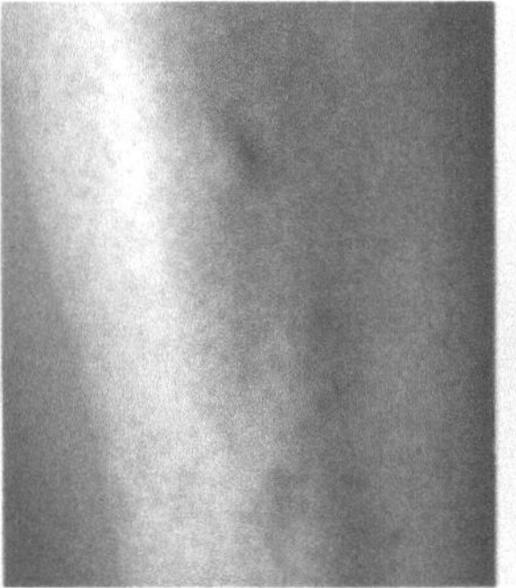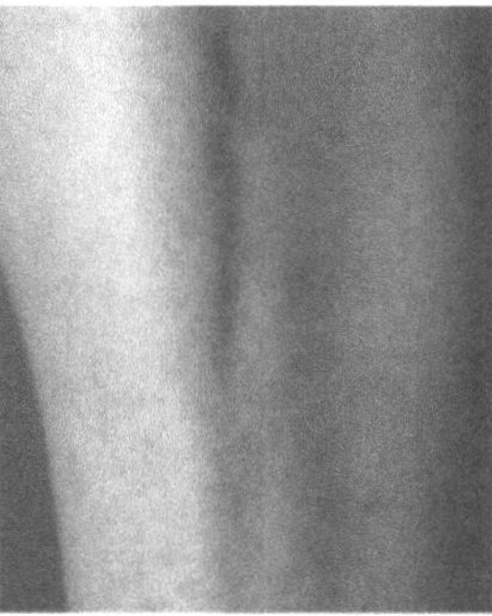

Figure 3.5 This patient came for consultation because of the single large "varicose vein" on her calf. The dark bulge appeared to be a fascial hernia whose diagnosis was confirmed by dosiflexion of the foot. Doppler examination could not detect blood within the bulge. Dissatisfied with the diagnosis, the patient had it operated elsewhere and to her dismay noted an immediate recurrence.

To perform the test the patient lies down. The leg is elevated to empty it of blood. To test reflux in the GSV, the SFJ is occluded with the finger, or a tight tourniquet is placed around the thigh to occlude the GSV. The patient then stands. If the varicose veins remain flattened for more than 25–30 s (the time required for the veins to be refilled from the arterial side) then their source of reflux must be from above the tourniquet, the SFJ.

If the varicose veins fill immediately upon dependency, they are fed by a source below the occlusion, possibly an incompetent perforating vein along the course of the GSV or the LSV. If the varicose veins do not fill immediately, the tourniquet or occlusion is released. Rapid filling of the varicosities confirms incompetence of the SFJ. A test showing the prevention of reflux with the tourniquet is shown in Fig. 3.6.

The LSV is tested by elevating the leg and placing a tourniquet just below the knee to occlude the LSV. The same maneuver is followed. The leg is lowered and the varicosities observed. Rapid filling suggests a lower source of reflux. Lack of filling followed by rapid filling upon release of tourniquet confirms LSV incompetence.

If there is a question about incompetence in both saphenous systems two tourniquets should be used. The LSV can be isolated by placing one tourniquet at knee level. The GSV can be securely obstructed here as it crosses the bony prominence of the tibia. The second tourniquet, placed below the flexion crease, then tests only the LSV.

From a practical standpoint the validity of Trendelen-burg testing must be questioned because the results are subject to many variables. For example, it is difficult to compress the saphenous veins in a fat leg. The saphenous may be occluded with the thumb or finger in the upper thigh but the transfer from lying to standing may cause the finger to slip and invalidate the test.

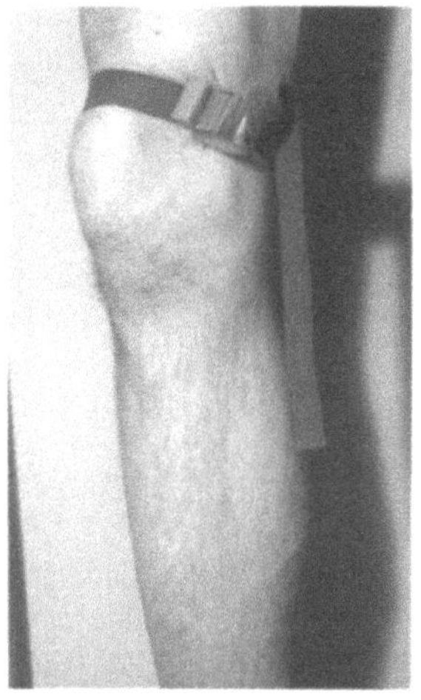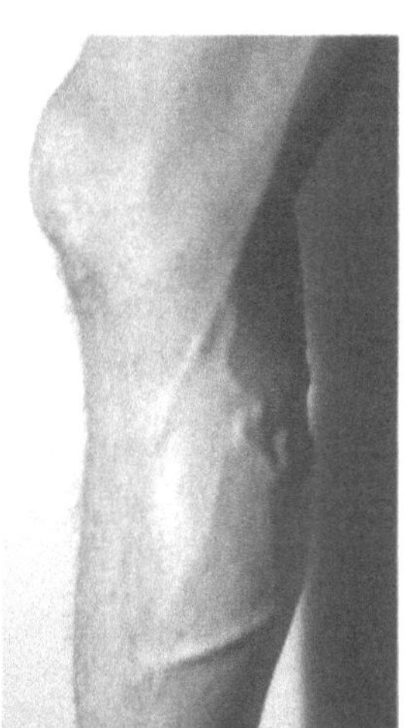

Figure 3.6 (Left) After the leg was elevated to empty its blood a tourniquet was attached at the knee where the greater saphenous vein (GSV) crosses the bony condyle. There was minimal filling during a minute whereas the blood rushed down the greater saphenous vein (GSV) when the tourniquet was removed. (Right) The GSV, the posterior arch vein and an intersaphenous branch to the lesser saphenous vein are obviously filled from above. The GSV is easy to compress in this thin leg but may not be occluded by the tourniquet in a larger or fatter leg.

The only site where tourniquet occlusion of the GSV can be assured is at the knee. Here the vein crosses the medial condyle of the tibia and lies superficially. At this location the tourniquet blocks reflux from any source above it. This would include reflux from an incompetent SFJ or from incompetent perforating veins in the mid thigh.

Fortunately Doppler testing has almost supplanted this test so that important treatment decisions need not be made on this test alone. Nevertheless tourniquets can be helpful in demonstrating to a patient that varicose veins are associated with proximal reflux and that obliterative treatment is important. It may also be helpful in testing for incompetent perforating veins below the knee.

Schwartz test

This test involves tapping or percussing the varicose system. It is mainly of historical interest, having been replaced by Doppler testing. The fingers of one hand are placed on the varicosities. Fingers of the other hand tap the SFJ or the SPJ sharply. If the valves are incompetent and the vein presents an open tube the percussion wave will be transmitted from the tapping fingers along the vein and be felt over the varices. [3] If the valves are competent and are holding the column of blood it is said that no pulse should be transmitted down the vein. This is not always true when a large but otherwise normal vein is tapped and a pulse may be transmitted.

A reverse Schwartz test places fingers over the junction and taps the varices. Reversing the ballottment in this fashion forces blood up the vein. However, its force too may be felt even when the valves are normal. The test is now of little clinical use.

Testing with ultrasound uses a similar approach. The technique of augmentation forces blood from a lower to a higher position. The lower leg or varices are squeezed, forcing blood upward. The squeezing hand is released and a Doppler probe determines whether there is reflux at the higher point.

Perthes test

This too is of historic interest. It was described in 1896 in conjunction with follow-up studies on the Trendelenburg operation. Perthes, an assistant to Trendelenburg, used it to determine whether superficial varices were a bypass for an obstructed deep venous system.

The varices on the leg were wrapped or tourniquets placed to occlude the superficial system. The patient was exercised to increase blood flow to the leg. If the deep system was patent then the increased blood could escape through it. If the deep veins were obstructed blood could not escape through the test-occluded superficial system and pain would develop as the muscles became engorged with blood. [4] The test in effect created venous claudication. Better methods are now available to determine patency of the deep system.

Pratt test

Wrapping is used to demonstrate incompetent perforating veins on a more selective basis than that of the Trendelenburg test. The leg is emptied and the saphenous vein blocked by a high tourniquet or wrap. The leg is wrapped to compress both saphenous trunk and incompetent perforator. The wrap is slowly removed from the bottom up or away from the site of a suspected perforating vein. Any filling of varices must be from incompetent perforators which have been unwrapped. [5] When testing with the Doppler a variation of this test is often used to isolate and identify incompetent perforating veins.

Valsalva test (maneuver)

Increasing the intra-abdominal pressure forces blood from the high pressure of the vena cava back into the femoral vein and possibly incompetent saphenous veins. A bruit or thrill can sometimes be felt in an incompetent SFJ. As a simple clinical test it is archaic.

Nevertheless the Valsalva test is regularly used as a test for reflux when testing with a Doppler or other ultrasound device. When positive, that is, when straining or coughing causes reflux, the test is considered positive. However, when no reflux occurs it does not necessarily mean that the saphenous vein is competent. There is a valve just proximal to the SFJ in many femoral veins. When the valve is present there may be no reflux in an otherwise incompetent saphenous vein simply because there is no blood to reflux as the upper valve closes.

Comments

Although non-invasive testing provides an enormous amount of information about the anatomy and hemodynamic functions of the venous system, a thorough historical review and physical examination is essential for a complete evaluation of the patient with venous disease.

References

1. Brodie M (1846) Lectures Illustrative of Various Subjects in Pathology and Surgery. Lecture VIII. On Varicose Veins and Ulcers of the Legs. Longmans, London, pp 157–164
2. Trendelenburg F (1891) Ueber die Unterbindung der Vena Saphena Magna Unterschenkelvaricen. Beitr Zur Klin Chir, Sieb Band. Laupp'schen, Tübingen
3. Brouse NL, Burnand KG, Lea Thomas M (1988) Diseases of the Veins: Pathology Diagnosis and Treatment. Edward Arnold, London
4. Perthes G (1895) Ueber die operation der unterschenkel-varicen nach Trendelenburg. Deutsch Medicin Wochenschr 16:253–257
5. Pratt GH (1941) Test for incompetent communicating branches in the surgical treatment of varicose veins. JAMA 117:100–101

CHAPTER 4

Venous Testing, Non-Invasive and Invasive

Traditional clinical testing is helpful in determining the general nature of venous problems. However, these techniques have become largely obsolete in today's practice of phlebology. Contemporary non-invasive testing methods provide precise information about the anatomic and physiologic changes found in venous disease. This knowledge in turn allows the clinician to make better judgments in planning appropriate, individualized treatment.

Generally two categories of information are required for the diagnosis and treatment of venous disease. First, one needs to know whether there is obstruction of venous outflow either by acute DVT or by chronic mechanical blockage of the veins and then where and to what degree there is venous reflux in the affected veins.

Traditionally intravenous venography has been the gold standard for evaluating anatomical changes, especially obstruction, in the venous system. Indeed it is excellent for defining the overall morphology of the leg veins but it has its limitations for evaluating the hemodynamics of venous function. It is still of use in some cases of suspected DVT and to determine collateral flow. Its use has continued in the UK and Europe, but, because of its inherent problems, non-invasive techniques are more popular in the USA.

Of major importance in the field of non-invasive testing has been the development of ultrasound technology. Both the anatomical and functional aspects of the vascular systems are immediately available to the clinician with this relatively simple, safe and reproducible testing method.

Non-invasive vascular testing: ultrasound

The use of ultrasound for determining blood flow depends on the Doppler principle, a physical effect familiar to every science student. Christian Johann Doppler, a physicist at the University of Vienna, described this phenomenon in the mid 19th century. He noted the apparent change in frequency of sound or light waves emitted or reflected from a moving object. A common example describes the increasing pitch of the locomotive as it approaches the listener and a decrease in pitch as it moves away.

When a moving interface, in our case red blood cells (RBCs), travels toward the ultrasound beam the reflected waves seemingly increase in frequency. The truth is of course that the frequency of transmission does not change but the waves are packed together as the object moves toward the beam of sound. Conversely the reflected frequency decreases as the blood moves away from the beam. The apparent change in frequency is called the *Doppler shift* and is proportional to the velocity of the moving blood. If there is no movement of the acoustic interface (the surface reflecting the ultrasound) or the interface is at right angles to the beam, there is no change of frequency between the transmitted and received signal and no movement is observed by the recording device.

For diagnostic purposes transcutaneous ultrasound is used to determine the anatomy and function of the venous system in the leg. Our hearing generally extends to sound up to 20 000 cycles/s (20 kHz). Ultrasound consists of those frequencies above 20 kHz.

Doppler ultrasound

Ultrasound is used in two ways for vascular testing. The most common use is to determine blood flow in the veins by a device called a Doppler. This technique is similar to sonar and radar and determines blood flow by measuring the differences between transmitted and reflected ultrasound waves.

Topographic anatomy is determined by the technique called ultrasonography. Two-dimensional images are produced and displayed on a television screen by analyzing the collected reflections of millions of ultrasound waves transmitted through the skin.

Most ultrasound instruments, whether Doppler or sonography, utilize a hand-held probe. The probe is fitted with piezoelectric crystals. When energized by an electric current, piezoelectric crystals vibrate creating sound waves. Ultrasound is generated by vibrating the crystals at appropriately high frequencies. In practice one or more crystals in the probe is electrically energized and becomes the ultrasound transmitter.

Conversely piezo crystals produce an electrical current when stimulated by an external force. Another set of crystals in the probe is designated as the receiver. As the ultrasound energy is transmitted through the tissue by the sending crystal some is dissipated, some refracted and some reflected back to the receiving crystal. The receiving crystal is excited by the reflected waves causing it to vibrate which in turn creates an electrical current. The current is processed by the instrument and reported in a variety of forms. Figure 4.1 shows the construction of a typical Doppler probe.

Most medical ultrasound devices generate frequencies in the range of 2–10 MHz, i.e. $2–10 \times 10^6$ cycles s^{-1}. The frequency used depends on the desired depth of penetration. The higher frequencies have less penetration than the shorter wave lengths.

Because sound waves are poorly transmitted through the air an aqueous coupling gel is placed on the skin and the probe placed in the gel for better penetration of the sound waves through the skin surface.

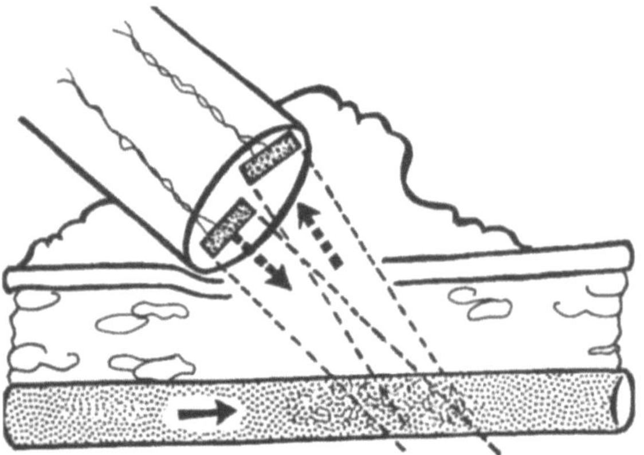

Figure 4.1 Piezo crystals send and receive ultrasound waves. The end of the probe is imbedded in a coupling gel to improve the transmission of the sound. An angle of 30–45 degrees allows the beams to determine the apparent shift in frequency of the moving blood.

Reflected ultrasound signals are processed by the instrument. The signal is represented acoustically and can be converted to an optical or graphic format. In this way the examiner can listen to the flow pattern on a loud speaker or with earphones, watch it on a screen or record it on a strip-printer for a permanent record. The process of examining a particular area of the blood vessel with the ultrasound beam is termed *insonation* or *interrogation*.

Continuous wave Doppler (CW)

Originally the device was known as the Doppler velocimeter. Currently the usual type of instrumentation is referred to as a CW Doppler. The ultrasound signal is transmitted continuously and reflected by any object moving in its pathway. The reflected signal is therefore non-specific and recognizes only the movement of blood. It will therefore report blood flow from more than one vessel lying in the path of the ultrasound beam.

Just as the radar gun in the police car determines the speed of your car the Doppler electronics determine the velocity of blood flowing in the vessel, usually expressed as cm s^{-1}.

Directional Doppler

Whereas the simplest Doppler device records only the velocity of the moving blood, a directional Doppler (some prefer the term 'bidirectional') instrument extracts information from the signal which determines the direction of flow in relation to the position of the probe. Blood is then represented as flowing toward or away from the probe. The directional instrument represents flow acoustically with stereo speakers or stereo headphones. One speaker represents forward flow and the other retrograde flow. When seen on a graph the flow pattern is either above or below a baseline depending on its direction.

Whatever the type of probe being used its ideal angle of incidence to the skin is 30–45 degrees. This angle permits the optimum reflection from the stream of moving RBCs. If the probe is placed perpendicular to the flow of blood it may not detect any change between transmitted and received signals because there is no shift of frequency. Commercial Doppler flow meters commonly have transducer probes with frequencies of 4–5 and 8–10 MHz. An 8 MHz probe is most sensitive at a depth of 2–3 cm from the skin surface and is used to examine the superficial veins. The 4 MHz probe penetrates to a depth of 3–5 cm and permits evaluation of the deeper venous system.

Information obtained from the currently available Doppler units record both velocity and direction of blood flow.

Characteristics of normal venous blood flow

When tested by continuous wave, directional Doppler, the wave forms of the superficial and deep venous systems demonstrate at least four typical characteristics:

- spontaneous flow
- phasic flow
- augmented flow
- ambulatory flow

Spontaneous flow

This phenomenon refers to flow heard with the Doppler while the patient is motionless and without compressive maneuvers by the examiner. It is heard most commonly in the deep venous system and is the result of *vis a tergo*, respiratory movements or local muscular activity. Spontaneous venous flow is more vigorous when the person is lying because upward flow is inhibited by gravity when the person is standing. In general the presence of spontaneous implies that the vein is patent and not obstructed. If blocked or obstructed the flow signal is not transmitted from the vena cava.

There is little or no spontaneous flow in the superficial system, at least when standing. One can hear spontaneous flow in the superficial systems at either saphenous junction but not usually in other portions. The presence of spontaneous flow signals in other parts of the superficial system suggests that one is hearing flow in the deep system through an incompetent perforating vein. Under normal circumstances venous blood flow is unidirectional, that is toward the heart.

Phasic flow

The spontaneous flow heard in a normal person is usually not at a steady rate but with a variation of velocity. Phasicity represents the natural variation created by respiratory activity, body position and intraabdominal and intrathoracic pressure changes as the blood moves from the legs into the vena cava. Breath holding or a Valsalva maneuver temporarily stops spontaneous flow to the heart for example.

Although flow may be phasic in character it is non-pulsatile when compared to arterial blood flow.

Augmentation

This characteristic implies the ability to increase or augment venous flow by compressing the veins. This maneuver is essential when examining the superficial venous system because the amount of spontaneous blood flow is minimal. As with all venous examinations augmentation helps determine patency as well as valvular competence of the veins.

Figure 4.2 shows representative tracings of spontaneous and phasic flow and augmented flow in the popliteal vein.

Ambulatory venous blood flow (AVF)

AVF is a characteristic which we have described as a result of work from our laboratory and is not a standard characteristic described elsewhere. Nevertheless the determination of normality or abnormality of the venous system depends on the alterations of flow and pressure resulting from exercise.

Exercise-induced blood flow was originally described by Bjordal using blood flow probes placed surgically around veins. [1] Although much of the data can be questioned because of the testing method it introduced the concept that there is active retrograde flow during exercise, a concept originated by Trendelenburg. [2]

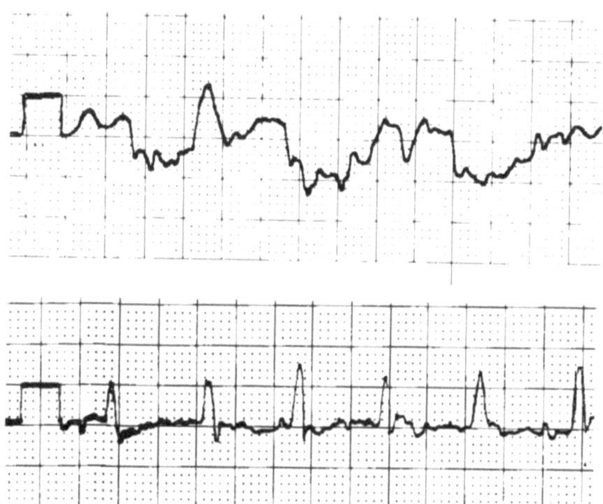

Figure 4.2 (Upper) This Doppler tracing shows both spontaneous and phasic flow in the popliteal vein. The patient was lying and breathing normally and the probe held as shown in Fig. 4.1. Blood was flowing spontaneously and in phase with the respiration. These characteristics could not be demonstrated with the patient standing. (Lower) With the patient standing the flow was augmented by squeezing and releasing the calf. There is rapid increase and decrease of velocity but no reflux. A momentary downward motion is seen as the valve closes.

The problem with any method of calculating ambulatory flow is to secure a measuring device over the vein. Tibbs introduced the concept of taping a small Doppler probe over the GSV. [3] Our laboratory has used a specially designed flat Doppler probe which is secured over the vein with tape or a self-adhesive strip. The probe monitors the continuous change in velocity and direction of flow during exercise.

Blood flow is quantified by measuring the cross-sectional area with the duplex scanner and multiplying area by velocity to obtain flow in ml s^{-1}. Although this method is open to error it is atraumatic and generally reproducible. It will be more fully illustrated in another section.

Venous Doppler examination

Every physician, having taken a thorough history and performing an adequate physical examination, should evaluate the venous blood flow using a CW Doppler. The Doppler is to the phlebologist what the stethoscope is to the cardiologist, only better. The examination is essential in determining the competence of the saphenous trunks, finding the highest point of reflux, the relationship of the two saphenous systems and testing the deep system as best one can. [4]

Technique

Every examination is performed to answer two basic questions: whether the veins are patent and whether there is reflux. A typical venous examination is shown in Fig. 4.3. Initially the examination is performed with the patient standing. In this position gravity assists the examiner by increasing retrograde flow when valves are incompetent.

The probe is first placed above the area to be compressed or augmented. A firm squeeze will push blood upward past the probe demonstrating patency of the vein.

The compressing hand is then relaxed. If the valves above the probe are competent there will be no retrograde blood flow and no signal heard by the Doppler. When the valves are incompetent reflux is immediate and a vivid Doppler signal is created. The strength of the signal depends on the amount and velocity of blood refluxing through the vein. This in turn depends of the size of the incompetent vein, the amount of augmented blood which can return from above and the space below the probe which can be filled.

A directional Doppler objectifies the reversal of

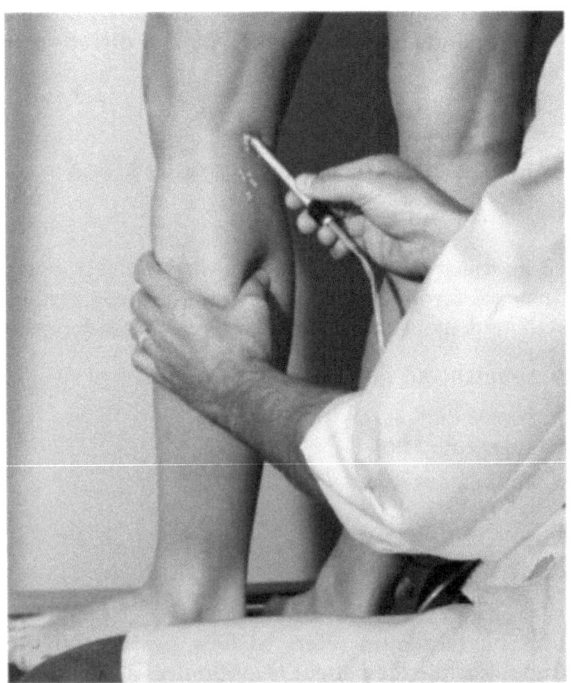

Figure 4.3 The examiner is testing the popliteal fossa by squeezing the lesser saphenous vein with the thumb. The gel path shows that the examination has proceeded from the ankle to the knee.

flow. That is, the dial or baseline shows the direction in which the blood is flowing. However, there is little question of the sound of reflux even when examining with a non-directional probe. The typical signal creates a to-and-fro sound which is easily identified after a little practice. This maneuver determines valvular competence. When the vein and its valves are normal there is simply no sound of flow after release of the compressing hand.

The augmentation maneuver is then repeated with the probe placed below the area to be augmented. The findings are then reversed. Squeezing should produce no signal if the valves are competent. In a normal situation the valves close and prevent retrograde flow. This valvular response is demonstrated in Fig. 4.4.

When the vein is competent decompression after release may cause a small upward flow to occur as the lower blood flows to fill the emptied veins above the probe. If the valves are faulty compression creates an immediate flow signal as blood is forced in all directions with no upward flow during decompression. Reflux continues during decompression.

After a complete venous Doppler examination with the patient standing, he is examined in the recumbent position wherein spontaneous flow is more easily identified. This suggests patency of the veins, especially the deep veins, since it represents blood flow from respiratory movements above the pelvis.

Augmentation maneuvers are again utilized.

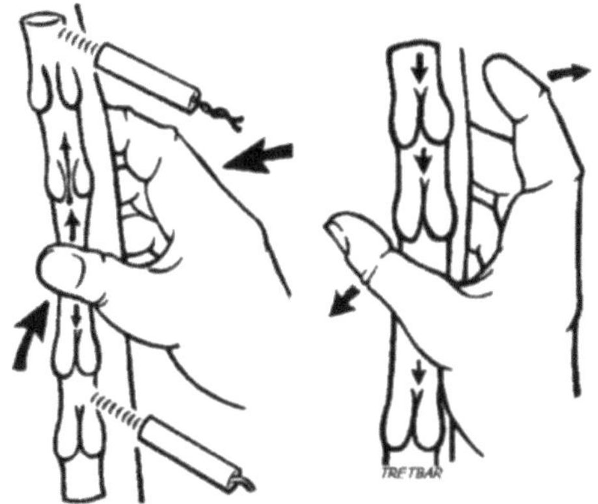

Figure 4.4 *(Left)* A rapid squeeze of a normal vein closes the valves below with no flow heard. Upward flow is heard above the probe. *(Right)* When the hand is released the upper valves close with no downward flow heard; the lower valves remain closed.

However, the demonstration of reflux is less definite since gravity does little to assist retrograde blood flow.

Greater saphenous vein

Examination of the GSV is performed with the patient standing, facing the examiner and with the leg rotated laterally. An 8 MHz probe is used. The examination may be initiated above or below the knee depending on the nature of the venous disease. If the examination is begun at the SFJ in the groin one should remember that the junction is much like the SPJ. There is a group of tributaries joining the saphenous or the femoral vein in a small area. Augmentation of the thigh or calf compresses a variety of veins including the femoral, the saphenous and either accessory saphenous vein. Incompetence of any one of them can be heard with augmentation if the probe is located over them rather than the trunk of the saphenous.

A couple of methods can be used to isolate the saphenous. Insonating the GSV a few centimeters below the junction and following it down the thigh will usually provide enough information to decide whether the junction is competent or not. Another approach is to augment the GSV individually. To do this it is necessary to isolate it from surrounding veins. The one place on the leg where it can be separated is at the knee. Here the GSV is superficial as it crosses the medial tibial condyle. It can be squeezed against the bone without compressing any other vein.

To try this maneuver acoustic gel is squeezed liberally down the medial thigh where the vein is anticipated. The GSV runs from a posterior position at the knee obliquely up the thigh to the femoral triangle. The clinician's left hand augments the patient's right vein and vice versa. The thumb compresses the GSV over the bone while the fingers are placed over

the patella for traction. It should be remembered that the vein is more posterior than one might expect, almost at the popliteal crease. Reaching between these two points may be a problem if the thigh is large or the hand small.

Unfortunately the volume of blood displaced by this augmentation maneuver is relatively small and only a small signal may be generated above the knee. The volume of blood increases as the probe rises on the thigh and the signal becomes stronger.

When there are varices on the medial part of the leg they are most likely derived from the LSV and can be used for augmentation. In many cases the highest variceal bulge is the connection of the varicose branch with the GSV trunk. The examination can then start just above the highest varix. Figure 4.5 illustrates how the Doppler probe is passed up or down the thigh following the path of the GSV.

When the GSV is incompetent and large varices are augmented there is a large volume of blood delivered upward. A large empty reservoir is likewise created, in which one hears a vigorous and prolonged reflux signal. There is little question of the status of saphenofemoral competence.

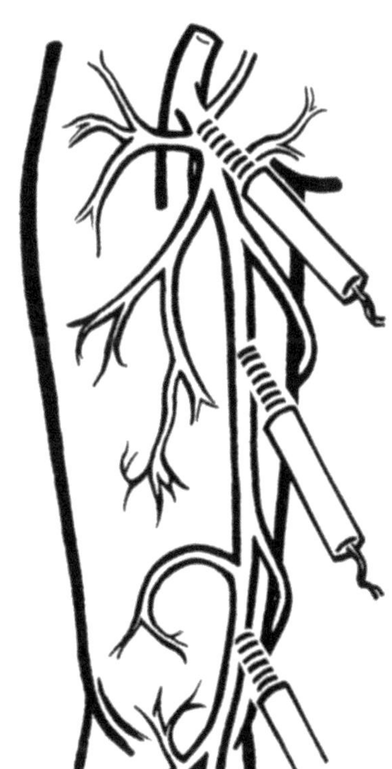

Figure 4.5 When the greater saphenous vein is examined the probe can start either at the saphenofemoral junction and move down the leg or it can start in the calf and move upward. The sound of refluxing blood varies depending on the position of the probe, the volume of refluxing blood and the strength of the augmenting hand.

In some cases the SFJ may be perfectly competent although truncal varicosities emanate from the GSV below the junction. Care should be taken to evaluate the entire length of GSV for other sources of reflux.

Incompetent perforating veins may reflux from the deep system into the saphenous system causing reflux below their point of entry. Unless the deep venous system is also incompetent there will be no reflux stimulated by a Valsalva maneuver since the vein is competent above the perforator.

It is not unusual to find vulvopudendal varices which have worked their way down the inner thigh to join the GSV in mid thigh. There is then reflux of the GSV at this junction to varices below. Apparently the continued reflux of blood from the pelvis dilates the GSV and a sequential incompetence develops until a side branch becomes varicose.

Augmentation of the varices can cause reflux to be heard in the perineal veins high in the thigh. Sometimes there will be flow from the pudendal vein tributaries at the SFJ which can be heard medial to the SFJ after forceful augmentation.

Occasionally both the GSV and LSV are competent but there are residual varicose side branches. A common example is that of varicose veins beginning in pregnancy. Apparently one of the saphenous trunks was incompetent during pregnancy and varices formed in branches along the course of the vein. Following delivery the saphenous became competent leaving the varices behind.

Even when grossly incompetent there is seldom spontaneous flow heard along the course of the GSV except at the SFJ itself. It is more evident when the patient is lying down. Patency of the GSV is not determined by spontaneous flow as it is with deep veins. However, spontaneous flow starting at a point below the SFJ may indicate the presence of an incompetent perforating vein.

Valsalva maneuver

The Valsalva maneuver is an attempt to markedly increase intra-abdominal venous pressure. Its effect on venous blood flow is then measured. It may be produced by a hearty cough or by holding the breath and straining as if to have a bowel movement. Some examiners attempt to quantify the test by blowing into a container with a measured pressure resistance. Others create a Valsalva by pressing on the abdomen especially when the patient is lying down.

To perform the test the probe is placed at the SFJ, along the course of the GSV or on the varices and the patient asked to strain. A positive Valsalva test is the demonstration of spontaneous retrograde flow. Reflux

can sometimes be heard the entire length of the vein and through its associated varices.

Valsalva testing is quite positive with varices deriving from vulvopudendal incompetence. Here the origin of venous hypertension and flow is within the pelvis, where a large volume of blood lies within the valveless pelvic veins. There is open communication between this source and the lower varices.

Many phlebologists believe that a positive Valsalva maneuver must be demonstrated for augmented reflux to be considered as significant. We do not agree. It is not necessary to demonstrate a positive Valsalva maneuver for reflux to be significant. There are a number of reasons for this viewpoint. If the patient has been standing for some time during his examination, the saphenous vein and its varicose branches may be completely filled with blood. There is then little or no room for more blood to reflux from the intra-abdominal veins.

Secondly there may be competent valves in the iliac veins just above the SFJ. Even with a totally incompetent saphenous system no blood will reflux when these protective valves prevent regurgitation into an otherwise incompetent GSV. Nevertheless reflux occurs during exercise or with augmentation because there is a large volume of blood passing up the femoral vein. Exercise decreases the pressure in the GSV and flow follows the path of least pressure, the GSV.

Common femoral vein

The superficial femoral vein within the thigh is not so easy to examine because of its deeper position. The principal finding in most cases is spontaneous flow. This is most easily heard in mid thigh on the medial side over Hunter's canal using a 4 MHz probe.

The common femoral vein is examined at the groin by finding the sounds of the femoral artery. The probe is directed slightly upward away from the SFJ. Spontaneous flow is easily heard here. Phasicity is also easily demonstrated as the flow varies greatly with respiration. Augmentation is created by first squeezing the calf and then the lower thigh. Generous flow is usually created with these compressions. Release should show little backward flow. However, if the probe is directed high enough and the patient is thin there may be considerable reflux heard. A certain percentage of iliac veins are valveless above the SFJ. This group includes those patients in whom a positive Valsalva test may be positive in the LSV.

The probe is then slowly moved medially and downward to find the SFJ then back to the femoral. Care should be taken when interpreting the sounds of reflux. The reflux sounds of an incompetent GSV may be interpreted as coming from the femoral or common iliac veins.

When there is a question of this sort, care should be taken to compress only the deep system. The saphenous system should remain full of blood and provide no space into which blood may reflux. Even then compression of a normal deep system can cause "overflow" reflux into an incompetent SFJ.

If there are varices in the upper thigh they should be augmented while listening to the SFJ. They may empty into one of the many tributaries entering the SFJ. The examination is then reversed. Gel fills the space between the end of the varices and the SFJ and the probe follows the sound of reflux, usually to the saphenous trunk or the SFJ.

Superficial femoral vein

Augmentation requires compression of the entire calf by the hand to empty the deep veins. A large leg can sometimes be a problem. An assistant may be needed to squeeze the calf with both hands. Above the knee the vein begins to twist around the femur and the probe may need less angling to get the best signal.

Calf compression generates a large flow of blood and a vigorous flow signal is generated when the veins are patent. If the vein is incompetent the reflux signal is also vigorous and clearly heard.

During the initial phases of examination small amounts of reflux can be heard in an otherwise normal femoral vein. This is caused by the sluggish closure of valves and is seen radiographically during venography. If this appears to be the case the patient should be asked to perform a couple of Valsalva maneuvers to close the valves. Then retest the system by repeating the augmentation from the calf muscles. If reflux sounds persist then it is probably genuine.

When augmentation is completed below the probe the femoral vein should be augmented above. This too may be quite a feat when the thigh is large. Assistance may be needed again. The vein is best squeezed on the medial side of the thigh in Hunter's canal. The GSV should be avoided by the compressing hand if possible, as flow within its lumen may be confusing.

On the thigh the squeeze and release should be rather quick and forceful. No sound is heard during compression if the valves are competent. A squeak or sharp barking sound is often heard during compression as the blood surges upward.

When incompetent, reflux is fairly easily distinguished. When the arterial signal is strong it may be confusing. Again augmentation may have to be synchronized with cardiac systole or diastole.

Varicose veins in the vicinity should be evaluated along with the larger trunks. While listening to the LSV the varicose veins are individually pressed or squeezed. If the varices are from the LSV, pressing the varix will cause reflux to be heard in the saphenous trunk.

Examination in prone position

When one is satisfied with the results of examination in the standing position the patient is tested while lying with the head elevated about 30 degrees. The findings at the groin and knee have been described. The femoral vein in the thigh should be re-examined if there is any question of competence. The major components not already examined are the deep veins of the foot. Only in the foot are the deep veins superficial enough to examine easily.

Posterior tibial veins

Behind and below the medial malleolus the pulse of the posterior tibial artery is quickly identified with the Doppler. The probe is moved until a strong arterial pulse is heard. It is directed upward. Venous flow is vigorous since the veins here are paired, venae comites. Augmentation is by squeezing the sole of the foot. As we have seen this compresses the deep venous arch, the foot pump, directing the blood upward. A strong signal suggests a patent venous system without obstruction. When the patient is lying there is little reflux demonstrated by relaxing the squeeze. Compressing the calf above the ankle probe will test for reflux. A normal vein will often show some reflux on initial squeezing. The calf should be compressed a number of times to close their valves. Continued reflux signals suggest deep venous insufficiency. This technique is shown in Fig. 4.6.

This testing can be helpful in and around areas of dermatosclerosis or ulceration to find incompetent perforating veins or connections to the deep veins.

Anterior tibial veins

Similar maneuvers are used to identify the anterior tibial artery and veins on the dorsum of the foot. These structures carry less blood than the posterior branches. Squeezing the foot sends little blood through the anterior vein although there should be some. The vein runs up the anterior compartment lateral to the tibia. Compression of the anterior compartment may cause some reflux even in a normal vein.

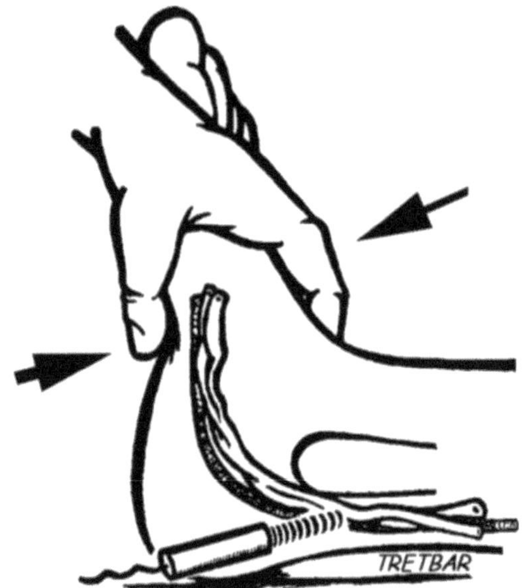

Figure 4.6 Testing the posterior tibial vein is simple. It is identified by its position next to the artery. It is easier to test in the upright position by having the patient sit with the leg dependent so that the plantar foot surface can be squeezed. The GSV can be easily tested in this sitting position as well.

Lesser saphenous vein

An 8 MHz probe is satisfactory for these relatively superficial veins. The patient faces away from the examiner. The knee is slightly bent (called the "Greek position" because Greek statues always have one knee bent) to relax the fascia overlying the deeper structures. Coupling gel is applied generously to the skin and the Doppler probe angled upward at 45 degrees. To avoid compressing the vein the probe barely touches the skin. Examination can begin either in mid calf along the course of the LSV or it may begin at the popliteal fossa. Usually the probe is first placed just below the flexion crease of the knee. Remember that the LSV runs between the heads of the gastrocnemius muscles but seems more lateral than expected. The LSV can be rather selectively squeezed with the thumb to augment it. While intermittently squeezing and releasing the calf the probe is moved back and forth seeking a signal of blood flow in the vein. Unless there are varices in the area whose reflux might be heard, it will be obvious when the vein is found. It can be followed down the calf, then up the calf to the popliteal fossa.

When the vein is competent the upward flow sounds like a series of squeaks or barks. This sound occurs because the volume of augmented blood is not great and velocity is high. Reflux is also easily heard with this maneuver. However, if there are adjacent varices it is not always so easy to identify the LSV itself as the flow signals become mixed. One may have to place the probe to the side and angle it inward, around or behind the varices.

As the LSV begins to turn inward to meet the popliteal vein the probe is tilted to adjust its angle. It may be perpendicular to the skin at this time. If the leg is not too thick an arterial signal is heard as the LSV approaches the popliteal vein which lies next to the artery. This approach is seen in Fig. 4.7. When both LSV and popliteal veins are competent the evaluation is not difficult. Following the flow sounds of the LSV up its course to the SPJ should be clear cut. Until the SPJ is approached there is no arterial sound to confuse the identity of the LSV.

When there is incompetence in this area, however, differentiation of source may become difficult. There are a number of veins which join together in the popliteal area, any one of which can give a reflux signal. The gastrocnemius veins often run between the LSV and the PV and join either vein in the popliteal space. The continuous wave Doppler cannot differentiate between these veins. It may be necessary simply to state that there is incompetence in this area or that there is incompetence in the distal LSV and investigate the area further with ultrasonography.

The position of the SPJ is of vital importance when surgical treatment is indicated. In many cases the SPJ can be accurately determined with the Doppler. This is true if only the LSV is incompetent. If there are

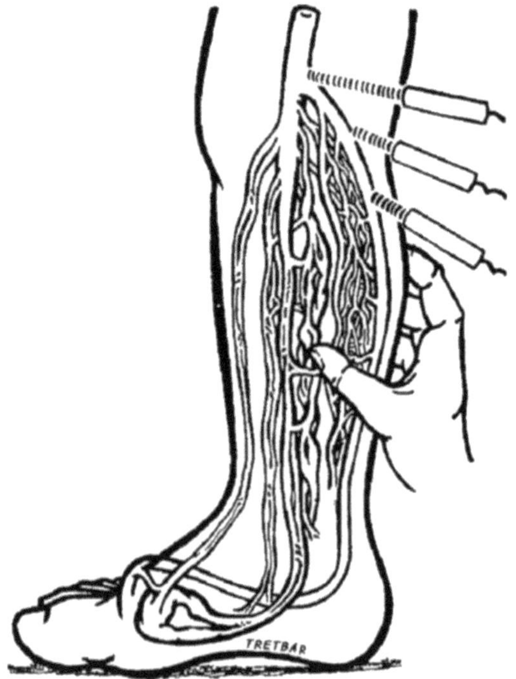

Figure 4.7 This diagram shows the method of evaluating the lesser saphenous vein from the lower calf upward. Either the calf muscles or the saphenous itself can be augmented. The angle of the probe changes as the vein curves inward.

other incompetent veins in the popliteal area the test is inconclusive.

To test for the SPJ the probe is slowly moved upward along the LSV as the vein is rapidly augmented. The probe is moved from a 45 to a 90 degree angle as the LSV curves deeply to approach the popliteal vein. An arterial signal should be avoided so that the popliteal vein itself is not insonated. When reflux is no longer detected and an arterial sound is heard the SPJ lies directly beneath the probe.

Generally the Valsalva maneuver is of little help in evaluating this area. Unless the entire femoral and popliteal system is incompetent there will be no retrograde blood flow with a Valsalva to test LSV competence. Incompetence is determined by augmentation maneuvers alone.

Popliteal vein

Once the relative position of the saphenopopliteal junction has been determined the popliteal vein can be examined above this site. To insonate the popliteal vein a 4 MHz probe may be needed for better penetration of the thigh. It is best positioned on the lateral side of the popliteal fossa and directed medially and upward. It is moved until the popliteal artery is located. The artery and vein lie side-by-side so that the arterial sound should be present at all times. Unfortunately the arterial pulse may confuse the beginner. Sometimes the venous sounds can be isolated by augmenting during diastole.

Initially the popliteal vein is checked for spontaneous flow. Ask the patient to breathe deeply and slowly. This generates the maximum amount of spontaneous flow. Unfortunately spontaneous flow may not always be heard when standing. This does not necessarily indicate an obstruction of the femoral vein. Care should be taken to check this finding when the patient is lying.

If flow is heard then ask the patient to stop breathing. The flow should stop. If it does not stop completely ask him to perform a Valsalva maneuver by holding his breath and bearing down. This should close any normal valves and stop the flow signal. On occasion a varicose vein may drain into an otherwise normal LSV. In this situation augmented blood from the varix will be heard flowing in the LSV but no reflux will be heard in it. These varices most likely originate from the GSV rather than the LSV. If on the other hand there is flow into an incompetent LSV the varicosis probably originates from the incompetent LSV. Care must be taken to isolate the trunk as completely as possible because varices overlying the trunk of the LSV may confuse the signal in the trunk itself.

Obtaining complete information in the popliteal area may require further evaluation with the duplex scanner.

Measuring reflux

Most phlebologists believe that reflux is significant when it lasts for more than 1 s on repeated augmentation testing. A strip recorder may be necessary to measure the duration of time. We will consider 0.5 s of reflux at the SFJ as significant if the reflux extends into the lower trunk and is associated with truncal varicosities.

To demand these precise definitions is misleading. The actual duration of reflux depends on the size of the incompetent saphenous vein and the size and position of the reservoir into which the augmented blood will reflux. [5]

For example, if a cluster of large varicosities is augmented into a large saphenous vein the resulting reflux will be both fast and short. There is little resistance to either upward or downward flow and a large amount of blood falls rapidly in the varicosities. If the vein is smaller with greater resistance it will take more time to refill the varicosities.

Alternatively, if the venous reservoir is small the refilling time will be shorter. A longer refilling time is always found when the calf muscles are augmented, there being a larger reservoir with greater resistance to flow. The Doppler printout of Fig. 4.8 shows these differences in response.

An attempt has been made to create a uniform method of augmentation. A pneumatic cuff is wrapped around the calf and inflated to a pressure between 80 and 100 mmHg. A large volume, rapid release valve empties the cuff in less than 0.3 s. This method augments both calf muscles and any varices in the

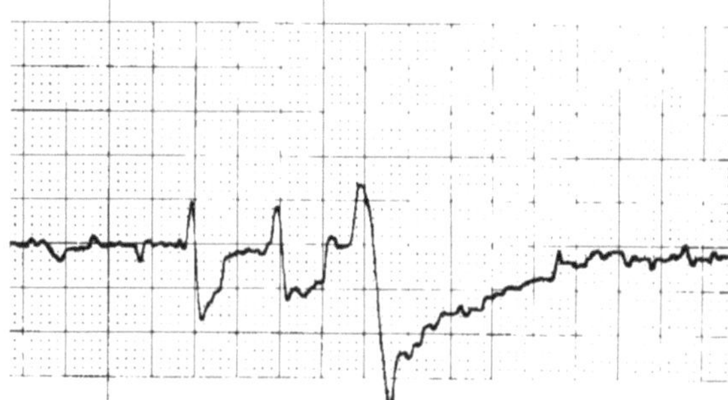

Figure 4.8 This Doppler tracing shows three reflux cycles obtained at the same site on the greater saphenous vein by augmentation of the calf. The first two cycles on the left show the result of a brief squeeze on a cluster of varicose veins; the reflux is less than a second in duration and of minimal velocity. The cycle on the right resulted from a hard, deep squeeze; the velocity is much greater and the duration is almost 4 s.

calf and eliminates most of the variations in augmentation technique.

Quantifying reflux

Many duplex scanners have software which will calculate mean blood flow in ml s^{-1}. To quantify venous blood flow the patient stands to maximize reflux. The duplex probe insonates the desired vein and the flow augmented. Augmentation can be either manual or by pneumatic cuff as described above. The pneumatic cuff helps to standardize the technique as much as possible. The software of the scanner will calculate blood flow in either direction. [6]

Interpreting Doppler findings

When the venous disease and reflux are purely superficial the findings are usually not difficult to interpret. However, deep venous insufficiency may confuse the findings by adding reflux sounds from incompetent perforating veins and other areas.

An incompetent GSV with branch varicosis is not so difficult to diagnose. Treatment plans can often be made from the Doppler findings alone. The same can be true of the LSV in many cases. With pure LSV incompetence the vein is easy to follow from mid calf into the popliteal fossa. Its junction is easily defined and no surrounding reflux sounds are heard. [4]

However, there may be more than one incompetent vein at the popliteal fossa and the Doppler cannot distinguish one from the other. There is usually a mixture of reflux signals of varying pitches and duration. When there is difficulty in clearly identifying the problem in the popliteal area a duplex scan is required.

The same rule holds true for any area of evaluation. If there is a question of the source of reflux or a possibility of outflow obstruction, other testing methods should be considered. Plethysmography, ultrasonography or venography may be necessary to fully evaluate the leg.

Exercise-induced blood flow

Although the method described above is the simplest way of quantifying reflux it does not reproduce the actual clinical condition of incompetent veins. That is to say the true significance of reflux is the degree to which it affects the venous bed during exercise.

Two major factors are responsible for the ultimate

effect on the leg. The first is the volume of venous blood which refluxes during exercise. The second is the ability of the various muscle pumps to evacuate the additional volume and thereby decrease venous pressure. The greater the retained volume the greater is the venous pressure.

Because it is almost impossible to hold the duplex probe over the vein during exercise another method has been developed in this laboratory to calculate superficial reflux volume during exercise. The method was introduced in Chap. 2.

First the cross-sectional area is determined with the duplex scanner. Then a flat, directional 8 MHz Doppler probe is secured over a superficial vein, e.g. the GSV in the low thigh. It can be taped in place or attached with Velcro straps so that it does not compress the vein. This technique is demonstrated in Fig. 4.9 on a patient with Klippel–Trenaunay syndrome.

The patient exercises is a standard manner, performing ten tip toes at a rate of one per second. This allows the results to be compared to those obtained with other exercise testing. The vein is rescanned to determine any change in diameter. If

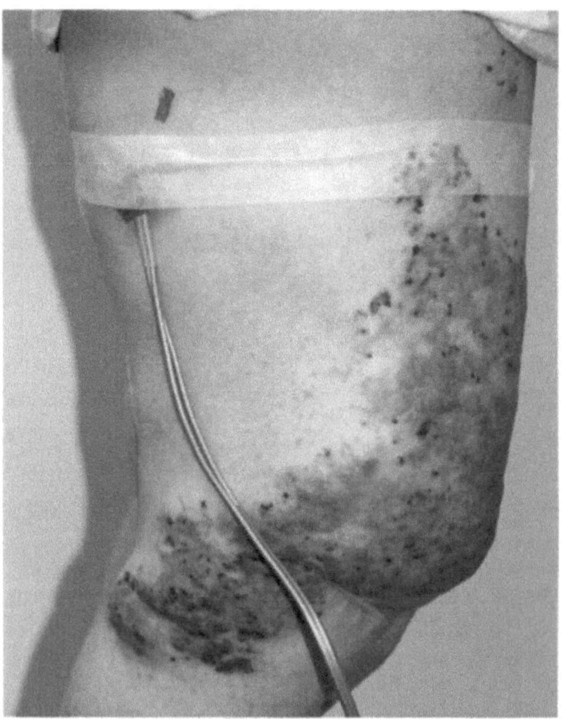

Figure 4.9 A flat Doppler probe has been taped over the vestigial lateral thigh vein. The vein was identified with the duplex scanner and marked. The patient was then exercised and a continuous reading obtained. The test showed slight upward flow during vigorous exercise. There was continuous reflux during light exercise which showed the effectiveness of the muscle pumps.

the scanner does not automatically determine cross-sectional area it can be calculated (area = πr^2).

In addition, the Doppler determines the velocity and direction of flow so that total flow is equal to velocity × area expressed in ml s^{-1} or ml min^{-1}.

The results of this testing technique are termed ambulatory venous blood flow (AVF). This then is an evaluation method which relies on exercise to determine the degree of reflux, just as ambulatory venous pressure measurements depend on exercise-induced changes in pressure.

The point is that the traditional augmentation method is a static evaluation, even when quantified, and depends on an arbitrary compression to determine reflux. It would seem logical to determine reflux individually in the condition which causes the problems related to reflux. Unfortunately it is almost impossible to measure flow in the deep system with this method.

Ambulatory venous blood flow findings

In the normal GSV there is an enormous variation of flow during exercise. Sometimes there is little flow and on other occasions the prograde flow is quite vigorous. When the patient with an incompetent GSV is exercised there may be a similar disparity of findings. Usually there is vigorous retrograde flow down the incompetent GSV during exercise.

This method of exercise testing has also been of use in patients with varicose saphenous trunks secondary to a DVT and in patients with congenital absence of deep veins. Here the question is whether the abnormal vein is acting as a bypass for the obstructed or absent deep vein.

Any such vein will show reflux with augmentation but if it is acting as a bypass there will be upward flow during exercise. Figure 4.10 illustrates a variety of responses to exercise using the flat Doppler seen in Fig. 4.9.

A comparison of the two methods, augmentation and exercise, has provided some interesting findings. For example, when augmentation-induced reflux is minimal to moderate there may be no reflux during exercise. In this situation the muscle pumps apparently keep up with the minor reflux so that the mean flow is zero.

Blood flow induced by augmentation provides useful information regarding valvular competence. However, it may not create an accurate picture of the true hemodynamics of reflux as seen from exercise-induced flow.

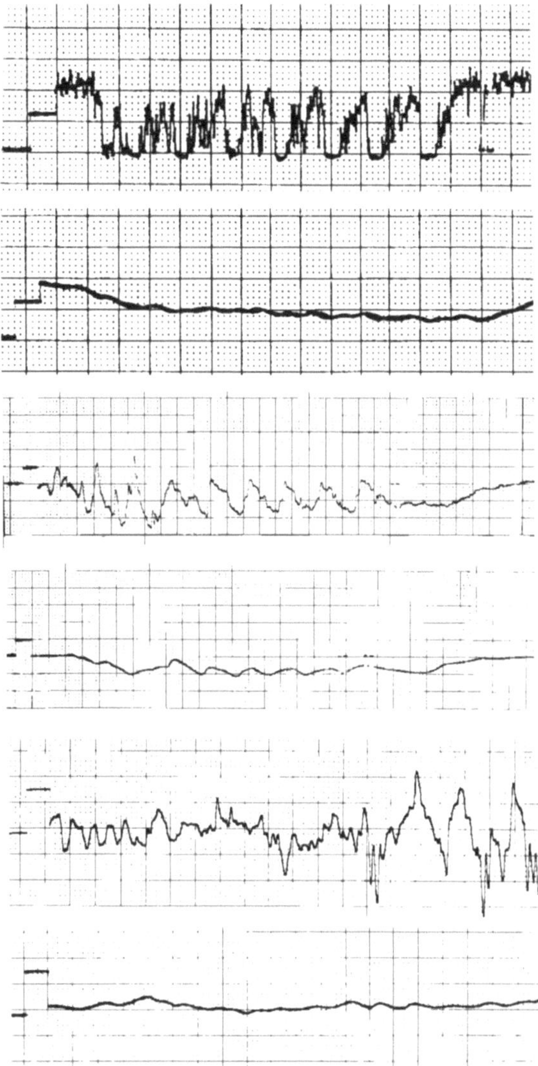

Figure 4.10 In these three sets of Doppler traces the upper of each pair of traces shows the actual continuous flow during exercise while the lower of the set shows the mean flow velocity. *(Upper pair)* This set of traces is from a normal subject. The top trace shows vigorous upward flow of blood with each step and the lower measures a velocity of about 8 cm s^{-1}. *(Middle pair)* These show continuous retrograde flow, reflux, during exercise in an incompetent greater saphenous vein. *(Lower pair)* These traces are from the patient with the Klippel–Trenaunay syndrome. The flow and reflux are quite apparent with each step; however, the muscle pumps are strong enough to maintain a slight upward mean flow. This test was made to try to determine whether the large lateral thigh vein and the huge hemangiomas could be treated or whether it was acting as a bypass for absent femoral veins.

Duplex ultrasonography

Although Doppler examination is the mainstay of venous evaluation and should be performed in every practicing clinician's office, the Doppler probe can only provide information about the velocity and direction of blood flow in an unseen vessel. In many cases this information is adequate to make an accurate diagnosis and to develop a treatment plan.

When more specific information about the venous anatomy and localization of reflux is needed "duplex scanning" is utilized. Ultrasonography, in the simplest terms, uses reflected ultrasound to create a visual image on a television screen of the tissues being examined. Rather than using a static beam of ultrasound like the Doppler probe, ultrasonography uses a scanner head which projects a series of ultrasound beams. The scanner head also contains the receiving crystals for the continuous output signal. The moving beam continuously scans the tissue, like a sonar, creating a slice of information about the underlying structures.

In former years intravenous venography was the gold standard for demonstrating the morphology and anatomical alterations of the venous system, especially for the diagnosis of DVT. Ultrasonography has in many instances replaced venography for evaluating anatomical and morphologic changes. It has the added advantage of providing hemodynamic information.

Currently ultrasonographic machines use "high resolution, real-time, B-mode, duplex" technology. The term high resolution is self explanatory. Real time means that the picture seen on the TV screen is a continuously updated image. B-mode describes the type of ultrasonographic technology which yields a two-dimensional picture of the field being scanned. [7]

The term "duplex" means that the machine performs two separate functions. The first is that just described, creating an anatomic picture. The second function allows hemodynamic evaluation to be performed in a point selected by the probe rather than the indiscriminate testing of the simple Doppler.

A specially designed Doppler is built into the scanner head. Technically the Doppler signal is "gated" as compared to the continuous wave form described in the previous paragraphs. It may be recalled that the continuous wave Doppler recognizes any blood flowing within its pathway. Gating the signal permits the Doppler to sample blood flow at any selected point along its pathway. In this fashion the appropriate vein is insonated, the Doppler signal placed selectively into it and its blood flow characteristics observed. The Doppler receiver is also directional so that the information derived demonstrates the direction as well as velocity of flow.

The newest form of ultrasonography adds color to the information system. Anatomical information in this system remains the same whereas the device converts the movement of blood into a colored signal.

Blood in the vessel is shown as red or blue depending on its direction of flow relative to the probe.

The technique of color imaging is similar to black and white. The scanning head is placed on the skin and the vascular area identified. Arterial flow, i.e. blood flowing toward the probe, is seen as red. Normal venous flow directed away from the probe is seen as blue. When the veins are augmented prograde venous flow continues to be seen as blue, but if there is reflux during decompression the color changes to red as flow direction reverses.

Either system, black and white or color, is admirably suited for examination of the arterial and venous systems. One non-invasive examination can provide both anatomic and functional information. This is particularly helpful when a simple Doppler evaluation is inconclusive or confused by a variety of refluxing vessels such as those found in the popliteal fossa. The duplex system allows each vein to be individually identified and its blood flow evaluated.

Because the data are digitized for display on a video screen the entire procedure can be recorded on video cassette. In many large vascular labs the technician records the examination which is later interpreted by the physician. The images can be recorded on photographic film as well. Recording also allows a later review when looking for other information than originally observed. Most units have provision for printing the video image as hard copy.

Indications for ultrasonography

Duplex scanning is useful in evaluating both the deep and the superficial venous systems. The superficial system is evaluated when the findings of Doppler examination are confusing or inconclusive. Duplex venous imaging is always indicated when DVT is suspected. When the clinical history, plethysmographic or Doppler findings suggest DVT complete duplex scanning of the legs and pelvis is mandatory. Repeat scanning is simple in following the course of DVT and for planning anticoagulant therapy. In the superficial venous system duplex imaging is useful in delineating the anatomy and flow of perforating veins, of junctional areas and especially the popliteal fossa. A definitive diagnosis is usually possible when Doppler examination is indecisive.

Methodology

When an anatomical examination is required the patient is usually scanned in the recumbent position with the trunk elevated 15–30 degrees. When reflux must be delineated it is advantageous to have the patient standing just as for the Doppler examination. The veins are first visualized in cross-section with the probe passed up and down the length of the vein. This visualizes the entire lumen of the vein when looking for a thrombus. Tributaries and branches are also well seen in this view. Longitudinal views then add information about thrombus extension. Performance of a duplex scan is shown in Fig. 4.11

Compression of the vein with the probe head helps determine the presence of clot in the veins. Veins filled with clots are incompressible. Patent veins are easily compressed and flattened. In many instances the valves can be seen floating in the vein lumen and their function evaluated. Physical measurements of the visualized structures can be made.

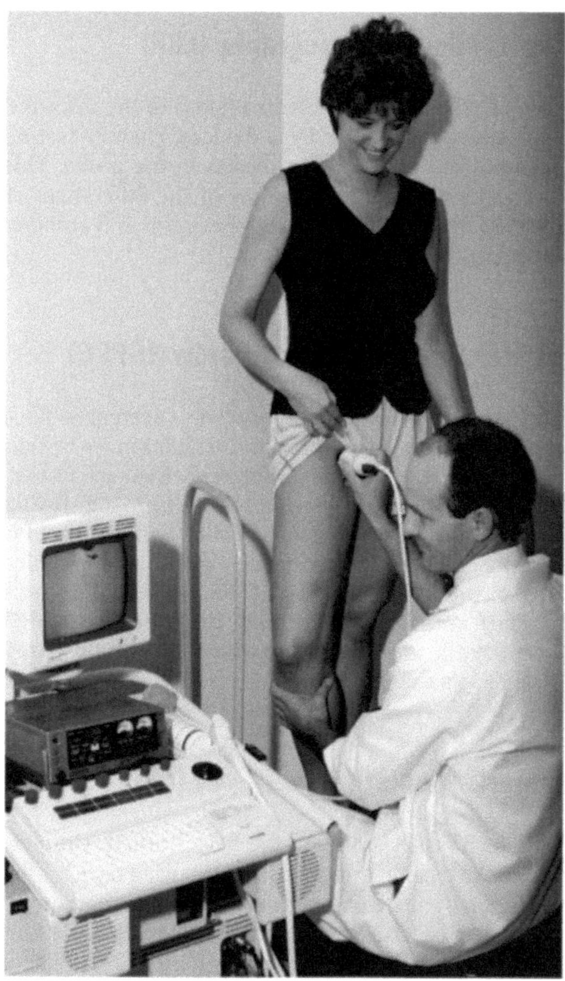

Figure 4.11 For functional testing the subject stands to increase the gravitational force in determining the presence of reflux. Here the saphenofemoral junction is evaluated. The vein is visualized, the gated Doppler probe placed precisely in the vein and the calf augmented.

When the physical characteristics of the veins have been determined flow functions are measured. As indicated the Doppler can be placed precisely on any vessel and blood flow measured. All of these determinations can be recorded on video.

Although many phlebologists are installing duplex scanners in their offices, the use of the scanner requires extensive experience. Therefore detailed instructions for the venous examination will not be provided here.

Plethysmography

Plethysmography describes a number of vascular testing techniques which measure changes in blood volume. Trendelenburg was one of the first to describe a true plethysmographic method of measuring blood volume.

In his monumental report of 1891 he tells of using a deep water bath to estimate the volume of blood contained within varicose veins. He first elevated the leg to empty its venous blood, pressed the saphenous junction shut with his thumb, inserted the leg into the water bath and then released the thumb. As the refluxing blood filled the varicose veins it displaced an equal volume of water. [2] This is identical to the method of foot volumetry which is described later.

Today the most commonly used plethysmographic technique is photoplethysmography. This is a semi-quantitative test for evaluating reflux in the microcirculation of the skin. The newest plethysmographic technique which provides a wealth of information on the macrocirculation is called air plethysmography.

Other testing methods – impedence plethysmography, strain gauge plethysmography, and phleborrheography – have been used for the detection of DVT and provide semi-quantitative information of blood flow through the deep veins. These testing methods have become largely obsolete with the advent of duplex scanning. Because the clinician may be using few of these tests in his office only brief descriptions of the methods are provided.

Photoplethysmography (PPG)

PPG is the most widely used of this group of tests. Basically it is a test of the venous microcirculation, a non-discriminating test for venous reflux in the small venules of the skin. The test measures the time required to refill the venous plexus after it has been emptied by exercise. Ordinarily it takes about 20–25 s for the arterioles to refill the venous capillary bed after it has been emptied. When there is venous insufficiency the plexus is refilled by venous reflux as well as arteriolar inflow. In this situation the refilling time is less than 20 s. It is held that the greater the venous insufficiency, the shorter the refilling time.

To perform the test a probe is attached with double-backed adhesive tape to the skin of the calf about 10 cm above the medial malleolus. The probe contains a tiny infra-red light and a receiver which measures the amount of light reflected from the RBCs. The patient sits with the heel touching the floor, and then activates the calf pump by dorsiflexing his foot ten times at 1 s intervals. A strip recorder shows an emptying during the exercise phase and refilling of the test area during rest. The refilling time is measured from the recording. If the refilling time is abnormal, usually considered less than 20 s, it represents a sign of venous insufficiency, although it does not determine the source of reflux.

A tourniquet is then placed to occlude the long saphenous vein at the knee and the test repeated. Should the test become normal with the GSV occluded it is considered the source of reflux. Should GSV occlusion fail to normalize the test it is repeated with the tourniquet occluding the lesser saphenous vein in the upper calf. A normalized test suggests pure LSV incompetence.

The results of PPG testing can be misleading if both LSV and GSV are incompetent. GSV occlusion may improve the PPG in this case but lower occlusion is necessary to normalize it.

If tourniquet testing fails to normalize the refilling time, two or three possible diagnoses are considered. It may signify the presence of incompetent perforating veins somewhere below the tourniquet. Usually incompetent perforating veins along the course of the GSV occur just above or below the knee and are occluded by the tourniquet and the PPG is normalized. However, there are other incompetent perforating veins which create an abnormal PPG. These may develop in the posterior arch (superficial posterior tibial) vein and be accompanied by venous ulcers of the ankle. Other perforating veins within the region of the short saphenous vein, gastrocnemius or soleus points, can also create an abnormal PPG with a normal deep venous system.

Failure to normalize with the tourniquet may indicate deep venous insufficiency. With an abnormal deep system there is continued reflux into the superficial system and the cutaneous venous plexus.

Our clinic's experience shows that when huge varices are present 10 dorsiflexions may not be able to empty this large reservoir. Tourniquet occlusion may improve the PPG refilling time but when the venous reservoir is still full the PPG remains abnormal. Appropriate treatment of the superficial varicose system reverses and normalizes the PPG.

Aberrations of PPG testing may also occur from a weakened calf muscle pump. Here a compromised pumping mechanism cannot remove the residual blood from a swollen leg or from varicose veins.

Arterial disease can also affect the results of the PPG test. Because the venous capillary is filled from the arterial capillary an alteration in arterial inflow can affect the venous refilling time. Arterial obstruction decreases inflow into the venous plexus. This means an increased venous refilling time according to the PPG test.

Like most testing methods the results of PPG testing must be correlated with other tests and clinical evaluation. It cannot become a definitive test for determining whether the varicose system should be treated nor should it be used as a sole determination of deep venous competence.

Light reflection rheography (LRR)

Because of various problems related to the infra-red light source in earlier PPG devices, current testing devices use light-emitting diodes in the probe. This system helps to eliminate some of the differences of the PPG test, e.g. variations of skin color and ambient temperature.

Digital photoplethysmography (D-PPG)

This method provides a more reliable system of PPG. It offers automatic calibration for differences in skin thickness and color and recalibrates before each testing. It can also provide continuous monitoring during continued exercise. Its use is similar to the other PPG systems; testing for saphenous vein incompetence with and without tourniquet, for perforator incompetence and for deep venous function. An added advantage is its compatibility with other computerized devices.

Impedance plethysmography (IPG)

This technique is one of the best studied, simplest and most reliable non-invasive screening tests for the detection of acute obstructing DVT in the iliofemoral veins. It is a classic example of venous occlusion plethysmography, a technique which measures changes in calf blood volume in response to the inflation of a proximal venous tourniquet. [8]

Because blood is a good electrical conductor IPG measures blood volume changes as a function of the change in electrical resistance (impedance) within the leg. The more blood there is in the leg, the lower is the resistance to the passage of an electrical current.

To perform the test, electrodes are placed on the calf and a tourniquet around the thigh. A high frequency, low amperage current is passed through the electrodes. No muscular or cardiac stimulation develops from the current. The patient must be at complete rest with the leg elevated on pillows. Venous occlusion is obtained by inflating the cuff to 50 mmHg, high enough to occlude the veins but not the arteries. The venous system is occluded for 2–3 min or until the venous pressure equals the tourniquet occlusion pressure and the veins are totally filled. The tourniquet is quickly released; in the normal condition the sequestered blood rapidly escapes.

The electrodes record changes in the electrical resistance which during this brief period of time are due to the changes in blood volume. Venous obstruction of the veins above the popliteal vein slows the rate of emptying. Generally a normal venous system will empty within 3 s. In most cases of DVT the decreased rate of venous outflow following occlusion reflects the degree of obstruction. The degree of filling may also be decreased if blockage has already impaired the ability to empty the leg of blood.

Depending on the laboratory and the cooperation of the patient, the test may be repeated four or five times to eliminate the variables and insure reliability. Usually a normal test represents an open, unobstructed outflow through the iliofemoral venous tract. However, an abnormal or equivocal finding may result from factors unrelated to DVT and the test must be repeated.

IPG is useful to determine outflow obstruction, presumably from an acute DVT above the knee. The results are immediate, objective and reproducible. A positive plethysmographic diagnosis of DVT in the upper leg suggests the need for anticoagulation, other necessary supportive measures and confirmation of the diagnosis by other measures. Traditionally intravenous venography was performed for verification. Now duplex ultrasonography has replaced venography in most medical settings for demonstration of DVT.

IPG is often used to follow the course of venous obstruction associated with high DVT and to test legs whose symptoms suggest recurrent DVT. Clinical signs and symptoms have never been useful in determining the evolution or course of DVT.

Phleborheography (PRG)

PRG is also called segmental air plethysmography, pulse wave recording or simply air plethysmography. To avoid confusion with the newer air plethysmography (APG, see below) the term PRG is used here.

Air-filled cuffs surround the leg and foot and measure segmental venous blood volume changes in response to respiratory movement and distal compression. The patient is tested in bed with the head elevated to distend the deep venous system. Six cuffs are applied. The highest encircles the thorax, essentially a polygraph, to record respiratory movement. Another cuff surrounds the thigh, three encircle the calf and a last one the foot. These are attached to a six-channel volume recorder. All of the cuffs record volume changes although the low calf and foot cuffs alternate to apply pressure to create an augmentation maneuver.

The PRG method depends on two blood flow phenomena; the first utilizes the fact that respiratory movement creates a rhythmic change in venous volume in the legs. Under normal conditions the cuff around the chest records respiratory movement while the leg cuffs record synchronous pressure changes in the leg and foot. The oscillatory movements are called "respiratory waves". A similar phenomenon of spontaneous blood flow can be heard in the deep veins during Doppler examination. Here the Doppler sound fluctuates with respiration and probably represents the same physiologic activity.

The second examination technique uses the augmentation principle wherein distal venous channels are compressed to create upward flow. After the cuffs are applied they are fitted to the leg by inflating them to a pressure of 10 mmHg. Calibration is obtained by removing 0.2 ml of air from each cuff. Respiratory wave forms are recorded as a baseline. Augmentation continues the test by intermittently squeezing the lowest calf and foot cuffs.

When an acute, proximal DVT blocks the flow of blood from the lower leg the respiratory waves are not transmitted from the abdomen. They appear to be damped on the tracing or are obliterated. Increased distal venous hypertension shows a non-phasic respiratory flow pattern. This is identical to the damped flow signal heard on Doppler examination.

Augmentation maneuvers normally show no change in proximal segmental pressure. The augmented blood volume is easily transmitted upward without pressure change. Obstruction may show a momentary increase since upward flow is blocked. From a clinical standpoint PRG is similar to other plethysmographic methods of detecting DVT. It is of little value in detecting small, scattered or non-occluding DVT in any part of the deep venous system. It may also be of little value in diagnosing recurrent DVT if flow has been re-established through collateralization.

Strain gauge plethysmography (SPG)

Not unlike impedance plethysmography, SPG evaluates changes in blood volume in the lower leg following venous occlusion in the thigh. The difference is that SPG calculates the venous volume by measuring changes in the diameter of the calf. The test assumes that the calf is circular in shape and that any acute change in its diameter reflects a change in venous volume. SPG is seldom used to detect acute DVT but more often to evaluate venous reflux and the general state of the venous outflow tract.

The original apparatus used a tiny mercury-filled tube attached to the upper calf. Electrical resistance within the column of mercury is proportional to its length. Volume changes within the calf alter its diameter and the associated length of the strain gauge tubing. Silastic tubing now replaces rubber and indium-gallium replaces mercury within the tubing. Even with this improved technology the use of SPG in the clinical setting is somewhat limited. Doppler and ultrasonography have largely replaced SPG as a source of dependable information.

Air plethysmography (APG)

APG is the newest of the plethysmographic methods to be thoroughly investigated. It measures absolute blood volume changes in the leg with the patient lying, standing and during exercise.

The device consists of a long air-filled cuff which surrounds the lower leg from ankle to knee. Changes reflected in the cuff are directly related to blood volume changes in the leg and are electronically calculated and recorded. Figure 4.12 shows the methodology for this examination.

The APG inflates the cuff to establish skin contact

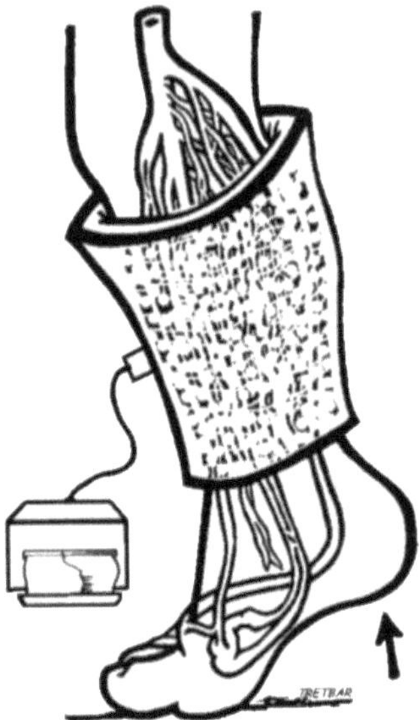

Figure 4.12 This diagram demonstrates the method of testing. The cuff has been calibrated and the subject now exercises to determine the change in volume caused by the muscular activity.

and to stabilize its position during exercise. Calibration is effected by removing 100 ml of air. With the patient recumbent the leg is elevated to empty it of venous blood. He then stands on the opposite leg while resting the test leg on the floor. The leg veins refill with blood and when full the cuff tracing plateaus. This change represents the functional venous volume. A venous filling index is calculated by dividing 90% of the total volume by 90% of the time required for complete filling. This calculation is a measure of the average filling rate of the veins expressed in ml s^{-1}.

One tip-toe is performed. The volume expelled with this maneuver is called the "ejection volume". Ten more tip-toe movements are performed to empty the calf veins as completely as possible. If the veins are not completely empty the remaining amount is recorded as the "residual venous volume". Appropriate ejection and residual volume fractions are calculated from these determinations.

Then, in a manner similar to that used in the PPG, an attempt is made to delineate deep from superficial venous insufficiency. The test is repeated with tourniquets applied first above and then below the knee. [6]

Proximal outflow obstruction is evaluated in a fashion similar to that used with the IPG. The patient lies with his leg elevated. A large thigh cuff is inflated to occlude and fill the lower leg's venous bed. After rapid deflation the volume and rate of venous emptying is calculated. Figure 4.13 illustrates a normal APG recording with the appropriate maneuvers needed to perform the test.

Arterial inflow can be tested during this maneuver for outflow obstruction. The initial rise in leg volume after venous occlusion indicates the arterial contribution to venous filling. As with the PPG testing, compromised arterial inflow can prolong venous refilling times.

Although the technique has some defects in calibration and reproducibility, comparative tests show that APG findings are similar to those obtained by invasive ambulatory venous pressure measurements. From the clinical standpoint this single non-invasive test evaluates numerous parameters of venous functions found in other plethysmographic methods. It can evaluate calf muscle pump function, the effect of superficial or deep venous reflux and outflow obstruction. In conclusion APG is a non-invasive method which promises to be safe, reliable and reproducible. Its findings of course must be correlated with the clinical examination and the results of other tests.

Foot volumetry (FV)

FV is a plethysmographic method wherein the plethysmograph is an open water-filled vessel into

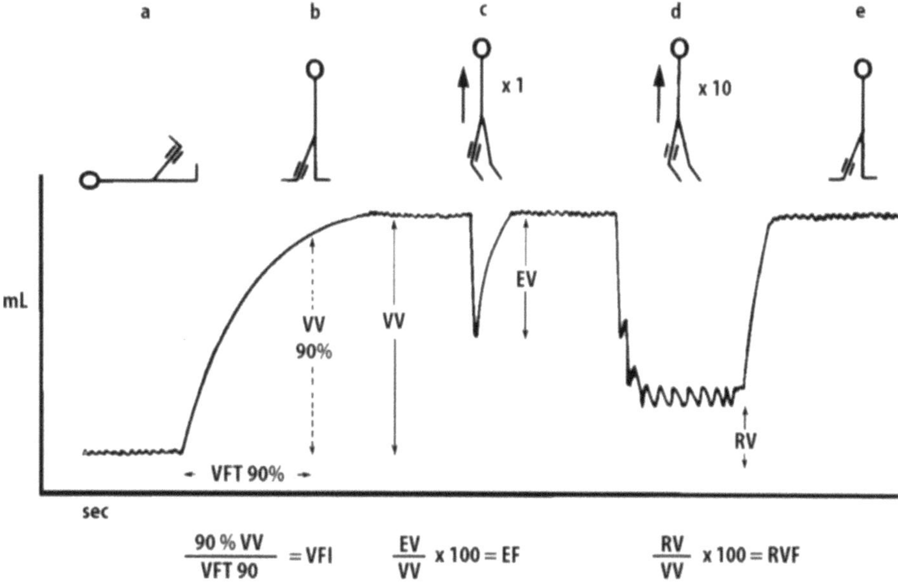

Figure 4.13 This is an APG tracing which shows typical changes observed with this method. When the patient changes his position from lying to standing (**a-b**) the emptied veins fill with blood and the cuff determines the total venous volume, "VV", which then provides a baseline for comparing volume changes resulting from exercise. It also measures the time required to fill the venous system, "VFT". This correlates well with venous refilling time as determined with ambulatory venous pressure measurements. One tiptoe (**c**) measures the ejection volume "EV", a test of muscle pump function. The system is allowed to refill between tests. The patient then performs ten tiptoes (similar to any plethysmographic test) to empty the veins as completely as possible. The residual volume remaining in the veins, "RV", is the difference between the maximum volume expelled and the previously determined venous volume. Calculations as shown give comparative mathematical indices. The residual volume fraction, "RVF", for example correlates in many cases with the ambulatory venous pressure.

which the patient places his foot. The leg is exercised by performing knee-bends. As the venous blood is expelled from the leg the water level falls. The change of water volume directly represents the volume of blood pumped from the leg. The refilling time can be equally well measured as the water level rises with the refilling of the venous bed. The method is illustrated in Fig. 4.14.

As with other plethysmographic methods tourniquets can be placed to differentiate between superficial and deep venous insufficiency. Although the volume changes correlate well with venous pressure changes, the information obtained with FV is probably more helpful in a qualitative way than a quantitative way. Although the test is simple and the apparatus inexpensive the technique has not enjoyed popularity in the USA. [9]

Magnetic resonance imaging (MRI)

MRI can be useful in a few circumstances where the venous system is involved in perivenous disease. Vascular tumors often entwine themselves around the arteries and veins. Computerized tomography, venography or arteriography may be necessary to define these unusual problems.

Thermography

This technique is used for the screening of patients with suspected DVT. The test assumes that DVT causes a temperature rise in the involved muscle mass with radiation to the surrounding tissues. The original system detected differences in skin temperature by measuring the infra-red emissions from the skin. The patient's leg was scanned with a camera which focused infra-red emissions onto a complex electronic detector. A television image was developed from the processed information. Unfortunately the telethermographic technique is expensive, sensitive to ambient temperature changes, immobile, time-consuming and not always accurate.

A simpler and cheaper temperature detection technique has been developed using liquid crystal technology. The crystals are embedded in a flexible membrane that is supported on a light, mobile frame. For the test the membrane is pressed against the leg in question. The other leg becomes the control. Liquid crystals change color in response to a difference in temperature. The result is a colored picture of the leg with a range of colors showing the variations of temperature on the leg. A built-in camera records the resulting picture.

An area which is "hotter" than the control leg

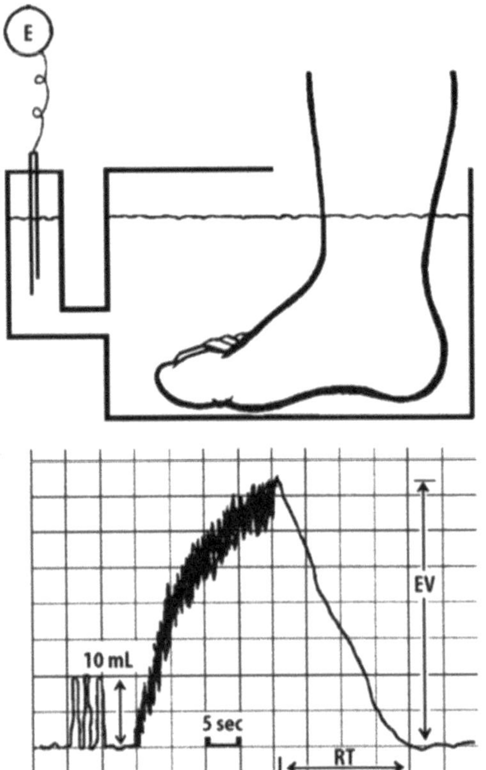

Figure 4.14 Foot volumetry is a relatively simple plethysmographic method. The foot bath is seen in the upper drawing. The graph below represents a normal test. The test is calibrated wherein each square represents 5 ml of blood. The tracing is similar to that seen with ambulatory pressure measurement and air plethysmography. Exercise gradually empties the veins and reaches a steady state. EV, ejected volume; RV, refilling time.

suggests a DVT. If there is no difference in temperature when compared to the normal leg, this suggests the absence of DVT. Varicose veins will show a smaller, localized hot spot but not the diffuse increase of temperature of a DVT. Negative tests by thermography find a high correlation with venography. In many institutions no further testing is performed if a negative thermographic test is found. It indicates no DVT or at least a DVT with minimal potential for embolization.

Thermography may be a useful screening test for suspected DVT or for those patients at risk of developing DVT. It is a non-selective test and one of several methods of detecting DVT; it should be correlated with other methods of evaluation.

Invasive vascular testing

Phlebography

Also known as intravenous venography, the opacification of the venous system by the injection of a dye has been the "gold standard" for the diagnosis of venous disease for the past 50 years. It has been particularly useful for the diagnosis of DVT. Although duplex scanning has largely replaced venography as a primary diagnostic tool in the USA, it is used for the confirmation of acute DVT and occasionally in follow-up. In Europe phlebography is still widely used as the primary investigational method. In many hospitals in the USA where ultrasonography is not available phlebography remains the only method of vascular testing.

Aside from image amplification, the most important advance in phlebography is the introduction of low osmolality contrast agents. These dyes are either non-ionic or dimeric in composition. Formerly the iodinated dyes were hyperosmolar and caused many side-effects. Nevertheless there are still occasional side-effects reported from the use of the newer dyes. For examination of the leg veins two types of venography are used, ascending and descending.

Ascending venography

With this method the dye is injected into a large peripheral vein, usually on the dorsum of the foot, and allowed to ascend to the pelvis. The customary technique has the patient's head elevated on a special X-ray tilt table while his weight is supported by the non-test leg. This position reduces possible calf contractions in the test leg which would pump the dye upward too quickly. It also allows maximum mixing of dye and blood which increases filling of the deep veins and minimizes possible artifacts. Usually a tourniquet is placed just above the ankle to force the dye into the deep venous system. Many radiologists prefer to watch the dye ascend without a tourniquet diverting the natural flow of blood.

A large-bore needle allows the contrast medium to be hand-injected using about 50 ml per leg. Television permits the radiologist to monitor the direction of blood flow and obtain serial films when the veins are optimally filled. Anterior–posterior films show the three stem veins of the calf. Lateral views may be needed for added detail and to visualize the muscular veins of the calf. Views of the femoral and iliac veins conclude the examination. Two sequential films visualize the calf veins in Fig. 4.15.

Valsalva's maneuver is applied as the dye reaches the knee. The valves in the femoral area are sluggish and may allow reflux until closed by the maneuver. This may also force dye into the deep femoral vein or the internal iliac vein as the dye reaches the pelvis.

The anatomical features of the veins and their valves are well outlined. Post-thrombotic changes can be

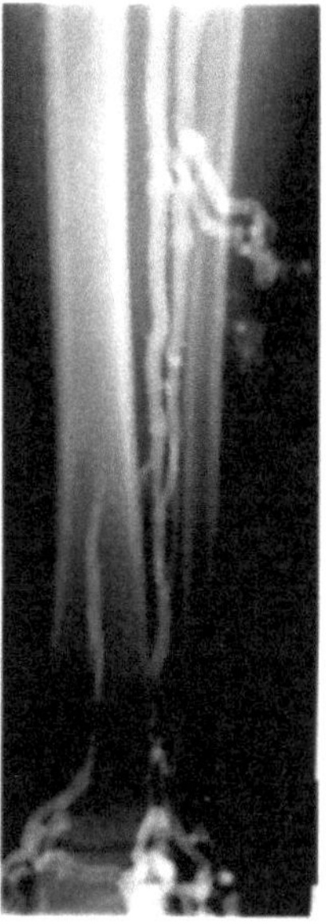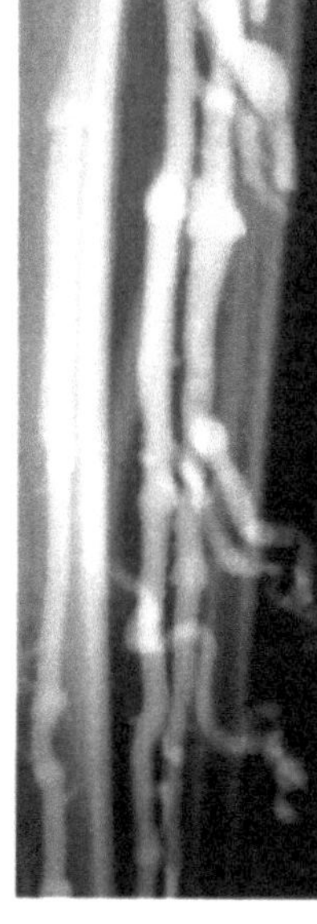

Figure 4.15 Ascending venography, often called "push phlebography", fills the calf veins. A tourniquet has been applied at the ankle to force the dye into the deep veins. In this manner a deep venous thrombosis can be visualized and incompetent perforating veins will be shown as they fill the superficial veins.

easily visualized with this technique as the dye sequesters in the valve cusps and refluxes through incompetent valves. Because the dye is diluted by the time it reaches the upper thigh little information can be gained from the long saphenous vein and its SFJ. [10] A different technique is required to visualize the pelvic veins, usually by introducing a needle or catheter into the femoral vein at the groin.

When descending venography is performed to confirm the presence of a DVT both limbs are usually studied. Thrombi are diagnosed when a filling defect appears persistently on more than one view of an opacified vein. The upper limits of the thrombus must be seen and as many veins identified as possible. The age of the clot and adherence to the vein wall must be estimated for proper treatment planning.

Descending venography

This method injects the contrast medium above the leg and visualizes its course as it runs slowly down the veins of the leg. Dye may be injected directly into the femoral or iliac vein by direct puncture. Usually it is introduced through a catheter inserted into the femoral vein of the opposite groin with the Seldinger technique. The catheter is guided across the iliac system to the other side. When pulmonary embolization from a DVT is suspected descending

venography may be performed through a more proximal catheter placed for pulmonary evaluation. Descending venography is especially helpful for evaluating the iliofemoral system and its pelvic tributaries. Pelvic and pudendal varices are easily seen with this method. These areas are poorly opacified using ascending venography due to the dilution of the dye.

With this method the SFJ is well opacified and reflux is easily identified. Reflux in the deep system and its perforating veins can also be assessed. However, DVT in the calf muscles may not be seen if the upper valvular system is competent and dye cannot be forced down the leg.

Varicography

With this technique contrast medium is injected directly into a varicose vein. The resulting X-ray shows the exact connections of the varicose system to the deep or superficial systems. It is a helpful technique when other testing methods fail to show these connections or when other testing methods are not available, e.g. ultrasonography. It is especially useful when surgical treatment of the short saphenous system is contemplated. The morphologic variations in this area are so great that an exact anatomic map is helpful.

Radioisotopes

Two other methods of assessing the venous system utilize the intravenous injection of a radioactive isotope.

Fibrinogen uptake test

This test relies on the fact that thrombi are metabolically active and that fibrinogen diffuses through the thrombus during its early life. The technique is thought to be the most sensitive method of detecting the development of thrombi and evaluating their rate of extension or dissolution.

[I^{125}]Fibrinogen is injected after thyroid suppression is obtained. The tagged material is identified and localized with an external scintillation counter. Because the fibrinogen is not rapidly excreted its deposition and position can be followed for more than a week. The legs are scanned daily and the results compared. [9] Because the test requires 24 h to establish a definite diagnosis of DVT it is used in a prospective fashion for patients at risk of developing DVT. So far its application has been mainly as a research tool to study the development, treatment and prophylaxis of DVT.

Isotope plethysmography

This is primarily a laboratory test which measures the blood volume in the calf by calculating the radioactivity of technetium-labeled RBCs. The RBC remains labeled for 2 h so that blood volume changes can be tested in any position with or without exercise. A scintillation counter attached to the calf records volume changes without the artifacts found in other plethysmographic methods. As a laboratory evaluation method it can measure calf pump efficiency, outflow obstruction and reflux in deep or superficial systems. At present it has little clinical value.

Ambulatory venous pressure (AVP)

This testing technique has already been described in Chap. 2. It remains the gold standard for determining the function of the calf muscle pump but has little value as a test for DVT. Other non-invasive tests, PPG and SPG, measure venous blood volume changes after exercise but report only indirect measurements. Other non-invasive tests have largely superseded direct invasive AVP testing in everyday clinical practice.

Lymphangioscintigraphy

When swelling of the leg appears to be lymphatic in origin the diagnosis is often made by a process of elimination. That is, vascular testing is performed to eliminate other primary causes of edematous swelling. If CVI is present this condition may be responsible for a secondary lymphatic problem. However, if there is no evidence of venous disease and the clinical findings are those of lymphedema no further investigation may be necessary to institute a program of lymphedema treatment. If there is a question about the condition of the lymphatic system further testing may be indicated.

Lymphangiograms are seldom used today. They required intravascular cannulation, the injection of an oily contrast medium and usually only opacified the regional lymph channels and nodes.

Lympangioscintigraphy injects radiolabeled human serum into the subcutaneous tissue between the first and second toes. It is quickly absorbed into the local

lymphatics and ascends the vessels as far as it can. In this manner it demonstrates the character of the vessels and blockage if present.

This testing is particularly effective in demonstrating congenital defects in lymphatic development or blockage by trauma or irradiation. [11] A typical scan is shown in Fig. 4.16.

Comments

In the USA non-invasive testing has largely replaced invasive testing, i.e. phlebography, as the standard for diagnosis of venous disease. Because it is non-invasive it can be used repetitively and its findings are reproducible. The equipment is portable, providing the opportunity to evaluate patients in their hospital rooms or in the outpatient setting. For the practicing phlebologist, the Doppler probe is probably more important than his stethoscope. Doppler units are affordable and readily portable.

In our practice perhaps 90% of all diagnoses are made and a treatment plan developed by the use of the directional Doppler alone. Although the smaller pocket instruments are quite accurate, evaluation of velocity and duration of flow curves requires an

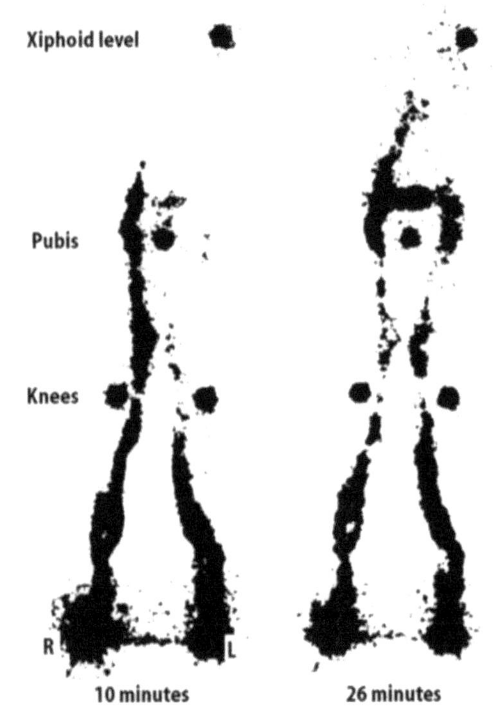

Figure 4.16 This lymphangioscintigram is a representative tracing and shows rapid filling of the lymphatic system. No blockage is demonstrated.

instrument fitted with a strip recorder. The use of the other testing modalities must be determined by experience and the needs of the patient.

References

1. Bjordal RJ (1972) Circulation patterns in incompetent perforating veins in the calf and in the saphenous system in primary varicose veins. Acta Chir Scand 138:251–255
2. Trendelenburg F (1891) Ueber die Unterbindung der Vena Saphena Magna Unterschenkelvaricen. Beitr zur Klin Chir, Sieb Band. Laupp'schen, Tübingen
3. Tibbs DJ (1992) Varicose veins and related disorders. Butterworth-Heinemann, Oxford
4. Schultz-Ehrenburg U, Hubner H-J (1989) Reflux Diagnosis with Doppler Ultrasound. Schattauer, Stuttgart
5. Vasdekis SN, Clarke GH, Nicolaides AN (1989) Quantification of venous reflux by means of duplex scanning. J Vasc Surg 10:670–677
6. van Bemmelen PS, Bergan JJ (1992) Quantitative Measurement of Venous Incompetence. RG Landes, Austin
7. Schadeck M (1994) Duplex and Phlebology. Gnocchi, Naples
8. Hull RD, Secker-Walker RH, Hirsh J (1985) The diagnosis of venous thrombosis in symptomatic patients. In Recent Advances in Blood Coagulation, Poller ed. Churchill Livingstone, London, pp 35–61
9. Brouse NL, Burnand KG, Lea Thomas M (1988) Diseases of the Veins. Pathology Diagnosis and Treatment. Edward Arnold, London
10. Hach W, Hach-Wunderle V (1997) Phlebography and Sonography of the Veins. Springer, Heidelberg
11. McNeil GC, Witte MH, Witte CL et al (1989) Whole-body lymphangioscintigraphy: preferred method for initial assessment of the peripheral lymphatic system. Radiology 172:495–502

CHAPTER 5

Patterns of Varicose Vein Development/Principles of Treatment

This chapter examines the common developmental patterns of superficial varicose veins, and describes the general principles for treating them.

Common patterns of varicose vein development

The common varicose veins seen bulging on the legs are usually dilated side branches of one of the saphenous veins. Whereas the saphenous trunks are thick-walled and contain a considerable amount of muscle, the side branches and tributaries are comparatively thin-walled. Continued volume overload and pressure may not affect the trunks but cause the side branches to dilate. As the wall of the vein dilates it also elongates. To reside in the same space they can bulge outward but must fold on themselves like an accordion to accommodate for the increased length. This explains the typical tortuous and serpiginous appearance.

GSV incompetence

The GSV is the usual culprit when larger varicose veins are found on the medial surface of the leg. Although its distribution is more regular than the LSV it nevertheless has a wide range of variations. It can duplicate itself, its side branches may come off at unusual points, it may dilate in unexpected places and may join with the LSV in creating a complex pattern of varicosities.

GSV varix

With long standing saphenous insufficiency individual varicose bulges will form at intervals along the saphenous trunk. Commonly a bulge is seen and felt in the femoral triangle near the inguinal crease. Although there is nothing particularly unusual or difficult about this problem many phlebology books gave much attention describing various differential diagnoses especially between inguinal and femoral hernias. Fortunately it is easily distinguished from a groin hernia by the presence of blood flow and reflux on Doppler examination.

The varix can measure as much as 2–3 cm in diameter and when removed is found to be a "blow-out", i.e. a dilation just below an incompetent valve. This varix is usually at the pre-terminal valve situated 5–6 cm below the SFJ. Many believe that the incompetent valve creates a jet of refluxing blood whose turbulence causes the dilation. Its formation is similar to that of a post-stenotic dilatation of an artery. Figure 5.1 shows a typical sub-valvular dilatation of the pre terminal valve at the SFJ.

A smaller varix is frequently found on the GSV in the low thigh as well. This bulge has often been described as the site of an incompetent perforating vein. My personal surgical experience is that few if any perforating veins reside beneath these bulges. They are usually a valvular blow-out as well. This particular valve is situated at the lower border of the superficial fascia where support from the fascia disappears. It may be the last valve protecting the lower GSV from reflux. Figure 3.2 shows a huge GSV which is varicose from the low thigh to the lower calf. It is this type of grossly dilated vein which is described by Trendelenburg.

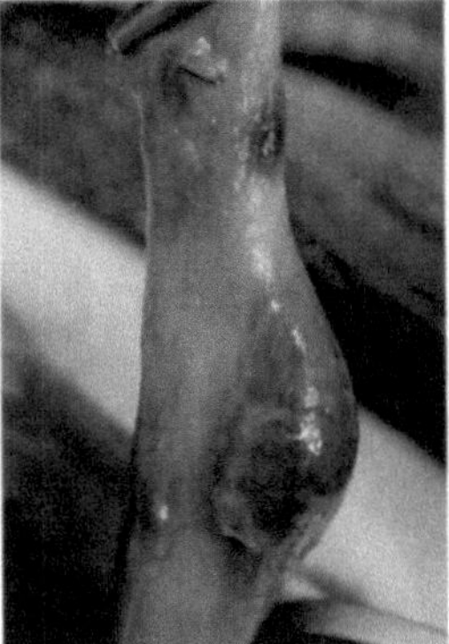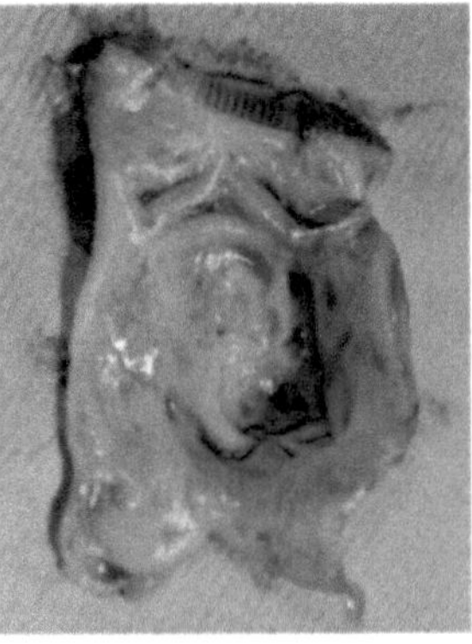

Figure 5.1 The photograph on the left shows a typical "varix" removed at surgery. The vague outline of the valve cusps can be seen above the dilatation. On the right the opened valve shows the valve leaflets to be atrophic and thickened. They remain open so that reflux from the femoral vein creates a jet of blood squirting past the leaflet. This turbulent flow then causes the vein wall to dilate below the valve.

Anterior lateral branch

The anterior lateral accessory saphenous vein is probably the most frequent site of varicosis. Clinically it may dilate to gigantic proportions, perhaps 2–3 cm in diameter. Hach describes two types of junctions. The *inguinal* junction with the GSV is just above or below the pre-terminal valve at the SFJ. In this configuration the vein runs from lateral thigh to the groin crease. In some cases it disappears 4–5 cm below the crease. The "iceberg" effect represents the "escape point" where the vein emerges though the superficial fascia. Its course is easily followed with the Doppler to the SFJ.

The *femoral* type runs more horizontally to join the GSF in mid thigh. When it runs directly upward from the lateral thigh it may join the lateral circumflex iliac vein.

An alternative pathway is to join with the lateral thigh and calf vein. Whatever its origin it can break forward at the knee to open the patellar (geniculate) branches over and below the knee. Here it can receive reflux from the GSV in the low thigh as well as from the SFJ. This combination of varicose veins is demonstrated in Fig. 5.2.

Posterior medial branch

Visible varicose veins in the medial thigh usually originate from the posterior medial accessory saphenous vein. Its origin is somewhat higher on the GSV than the anterior lateral branch often from 8–10 cm distal to the saphenous junction. In most cases the branches are deeper than the anterior branches and when incompetent the varices may not become

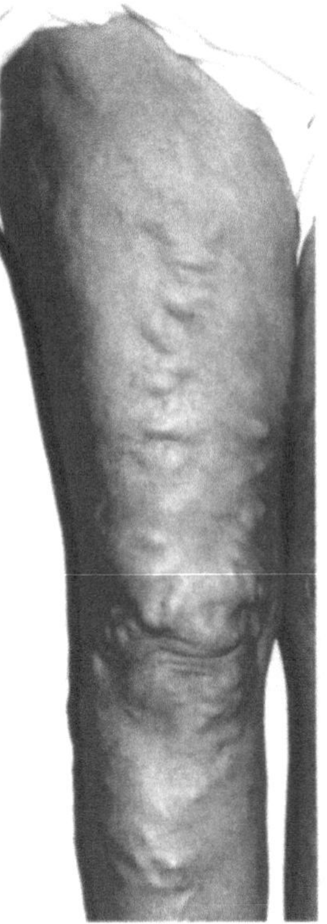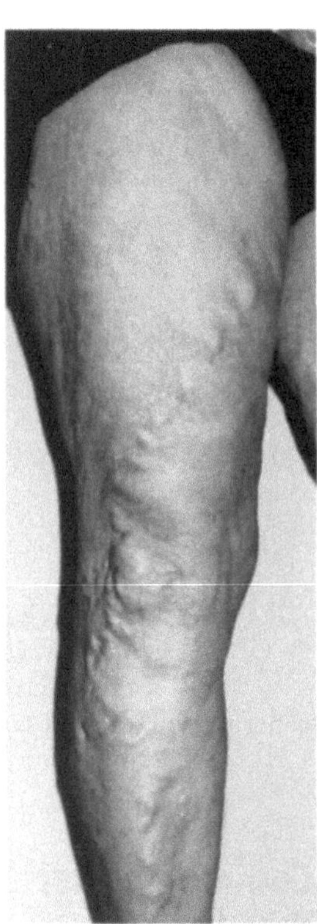

Figure 5.2 These photographs demonstrate the two types of attachment of the anterior lateral vein. On the left the *inguinal* junction is well seen. The varicose condition is well advanced so that other varicosities have formed as well. The *femoral* attachment is seen on the right. Both types may run over or around the knee to join the calf veins.

apparent until they reach the posterior thigh. Here the typical subcutaneous varicose pattern involves the posterior thigh vein running across to the lateral thigh and down to the upper calf. A Doppler examination again traces the varicose posterior thigh vein upward to the GSV or the SFJ. Figure 5.3 shows the high thigh attachment in an unusually thin patient.

Mid thigh vein

Sometimes it seems that the GSV becomes varicose in the mid thigh. When visualized by ultrasonography this dilated vein is usually a distinct branch arising from and running parallel to the LSV. It represents a true duplication of the LSV, an event which is more common than thought. When smaller it probably is a branch of the GSV. Below the knee it joins with the anterior or posterior arch veins where it often forms clusters of varicosities. It can also run posteriorly to join the intersaphenous tributary causing varicose veins which drain into the LSV.

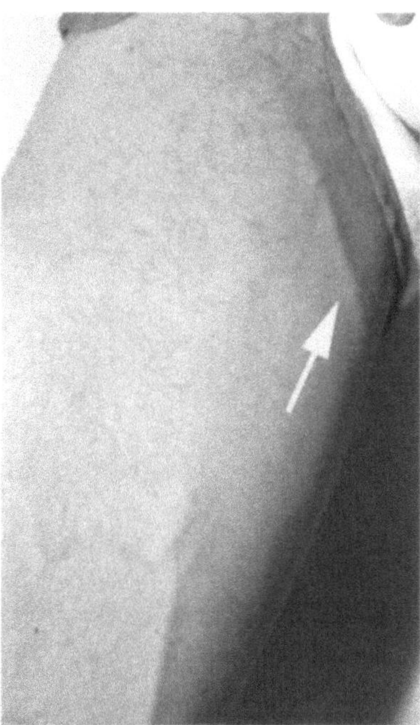

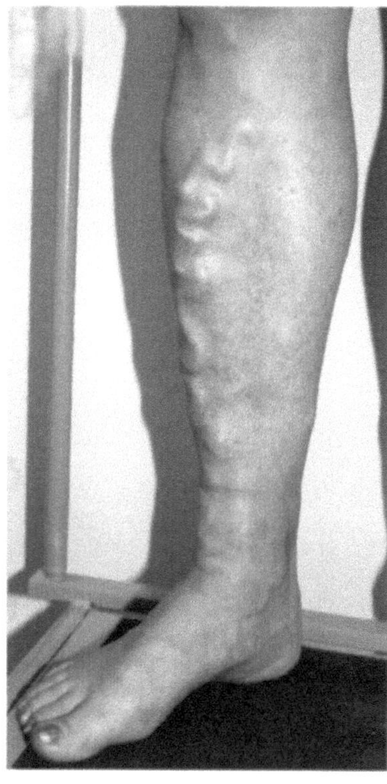

Figure 5.3 The arrow points to the posterior medial branch which is unusually visible. Usually it runs more deeply than the anterior branch and may remain in a subfascial position in the posterior thigh. The greater saphenous vein is dilated in mid thigh and gives off a dilated anterior branch.

Anterior arch vein

In our practice the anterior arch vein is more commonly affected by GSV insufficiency than the posterior arch vein. The anterior branch is far more visible because it runs over the tibia as it ascends from the dorsal arch vein in the foot. Although there are small perforating veins which connect it with the deeper anterior tibial veins they seldom participate in the development of varicosis. Varicose arch veins are frequently intertwined with varicose patellar or lateral thigh branches. A typical varicose anterior arch vein is shown in Fig. 5.4.

Posterior arch vein

The posterior arch vein has always fascinated the anatomist and phlebologist. It is sometimes called Leonardo's vein, having been seen among da Vinci's anatomic drawings. It overlies the deep posterior tibial veins and communicates through Cockett's and Sherman's perforating veins. This position has implicated the veins in the development of venous ulcers which are usually found in this region.

Clinically varicose posterior arch veins wander around the medial and posterior calf and may share a common saphenous branch with the anterior group.

Figure 5.4 Here the varicose anterior arch vein is the only evidence of an incompetent greater saphenous vein. It is one of the most common saphenous branches affected by venous hypertension but may also be prominent, even when normal, as it crosses over the tibia.

Many phlebologists contend that local GSV perforator incompetence, e.g. Boyd's, is a common cause of reflux and varicosis in this area. It is my practice to remove saphenous blebs or a short segment of GSV at the knee when these branches are varicose. Seldom have I found Boyd's perforating vein to be incompetent. Nevertheless when there is local GSV incompetence with a normal SFJ this cause should be considered. Figure 5.5 illustrates a varicose posterior arch vein emanating from a dilated GSV.

LSV incompetence

Just as the LSV itself is variable the truncal varices deriving from LSV incompetence are more variable than those from the GSV. Varicosities originate from all levels of the vein and can cluster above or below the flexion crease of the knee. They extend laterally or bunch up medially often connecting with branches of the GSV, especially the posterior arch vein and patellar branches.

A common diagnostic problem occurs when varices on the posterior leg overlie the popliteal fossa. There is such widespread reflux that a diagnosis with the

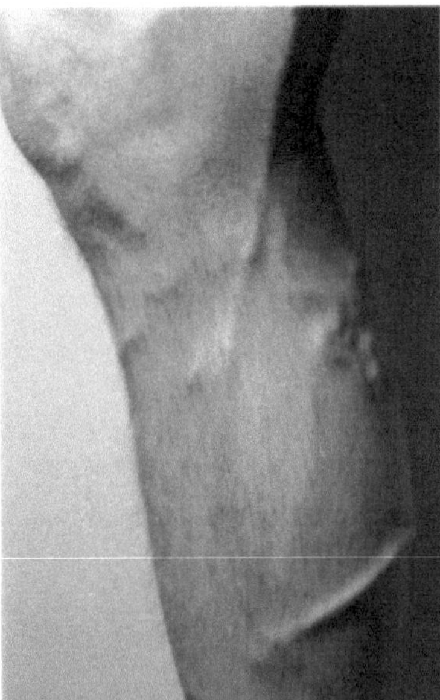

Figure 5.5 In this patient, also seen in Fig. 5.3, the greater saphenous vein (GSV) and all of its side branches are incompetent and grossly dilated. Although the posterior arch vein is frequently varicose its attachment to the GSV is not normally so apparent. Just below its junction is an incompetent anterior arch vein. In mid calf a large intersaphenous branch is seen joining the GSV and the lesser saphenous vein.

Doppler alone may be impossible. In this case ultrasonography is necessary to evaluate the integrity of the LSV and to establish the primary source of reflux.

For the surgeon ultrasonography will establish the exact site of the SPJ and determine whether the tributaries of the gastrocnemius join the LSV or popliteal vein. A large mass of varicose veins is shown in Fig. 5.6 coming directly from an incompetent LSV.

Foot veins

There may be varicosities anywhere in the foot as a result of GSV or LSV incompetence. By the time the varicose condition reaches the foot the entire complex of foot veins may be affected.

When varicose veins run all the way down the leg from thigh or calf to the foot we assume they all derive from an incompetent saphenous vein. A simple clinical test challenges this opinion in some cases. When the patient is standing varices of the leg and foot bulge equally. However, when the patient lies down all of the varicosities flatten except those on the foot. Gradual elevation of the leg finally flattens the varices. This clinical test demonstrates that the foot veins are under a higher pressure system than those of the upper leg. One explanation is that the veins are arterialized.

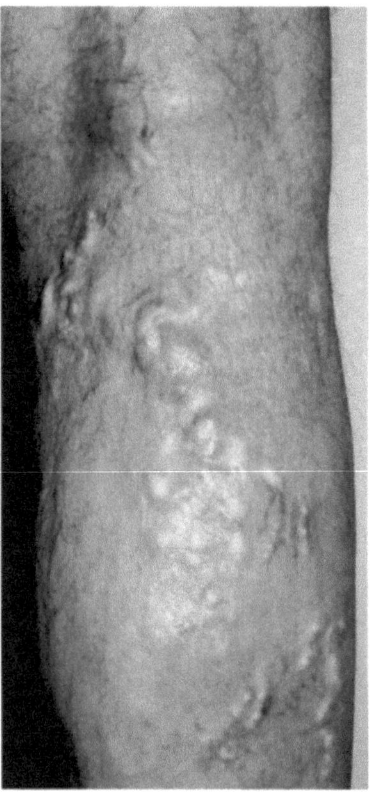

Figure 5.6 Ultrasound demonstrated that these varicosities arose solely from the incompetent lesser saphenous vein (LSV). Care must be taken to assess both saphenous systems because similar varices can develop from the greater saphenous vein (GSV). Venous hypertension can be transmitted from the GSV through the intersaphenous connecting veins to the veins of the posterior calf. Occasionally the LSV will be rendered incompetent by the same process.

Blood observed at surgery is noticeably redder in some of them. The foot veins are also tougher with thicker muscular walls than one might expect.

When the varices are removed surgically one may also find small perforating veins, usually on the medial aspect of the ankle, the inframalleolar perforator, associated with the varices.

Non-saphenous veins

Varicose veins which are not derived from incompetent saphenous trunks are usually smaller, under less pressure and more readily treated with injection sclerotherapy.

Vulvopudendal veins

Incompetent vulval and pudendal veins are an exception to this rule. Because they originate in the pelvis or higher gonadal veins they can be a source of considerable venous hypertension with rather exuberant secondary varices. From a phlebologic viewpoint it is almost impossible to empty them with exercise. Therefore the ambulatory pressure remains high.

A review of some 80 patients treated in our clinic for vulvopudendal varicosities showed three general patterns of presentation. They all show a cluster of small to large varices in the posterior triangle behind the adductor muscle below the labia and coming directly from the perineum. Although this may be the only involved area they usually attach themselves to lower veins. This cluster of high thigh veins is represented in Fig. 5.7.

The first common attachment is to the GSV at mid thigh. Here the reflux from the pelvis can distend the distal GSV rendering it incompetent. The situation may be perplexing to the examiner. The varicose veins seem to be typical for GSV incompetence although the proximal GSV and SFJ are normal on Doppler examination. The veins connecting the pudendal and GSV may not be visible but can be traced with the Doppler or ultrasonography.

These pudendal veins may be the sole cause of saphenous varices springing from the GSV. In most cases treating the pudendal veins controls the pressure

source to the GSV with subsequent shrinkage and restoration of competence. The distal varices are treated in the usual fashion.

An alternative pathway of the pudendal veins is to join the posterior medial GSV branch as it passes to the posterior thigh. The GSV and SFJ are again normal in this situation. A typical formation is the varicose posterior lateral thigh vein. There may be associated varicosities running along the gluteal fold or even on the buttocks. Injection sclerotherapy is useful when there is clustering of veins although large pudendal trunks can be successfully phlebectomized.

Posterior lateral thigh veins

Commonly the posterior medial branch of the GSV or varicose pudendal veins break into the superficial veins of the posterior and lateral thigh. Fig. 5.8 shows this typical pattern of varices.

An alternative, however, shows the posterior thigh to be free of varicosis whereas the varicose system is situated only on the lateral thigh and calf veins. When present they are usually smaller than those seen in Fig. 5.8. Recent work shows that the venous hypertension responsible for their dilatation may originate from small incompetent perforating veins arising from the peroneal veins around the fibular head. [1]

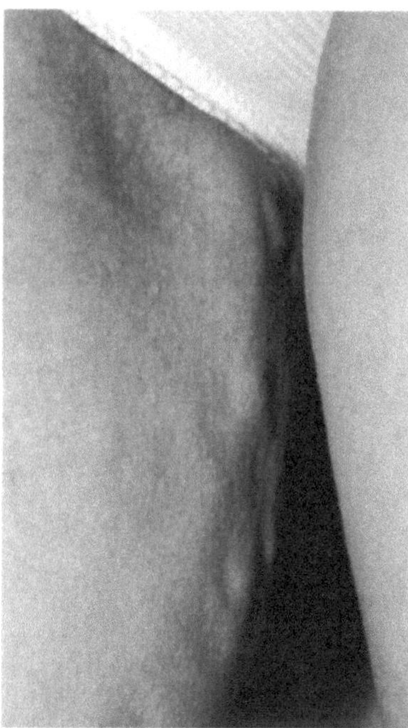

Figure 5.7 These vulvopudendal varices developed after two pregnancies and are quite symptomatic before her period. They arise in the posterior triangle which is present behind the adductor muscles. In this photograph the concavity of the anterior (femoral) triangle is equally visible. Because varicose pudendal veins are not always so apparent they should be sought for when there are complaints of pelvic or thigh pain.

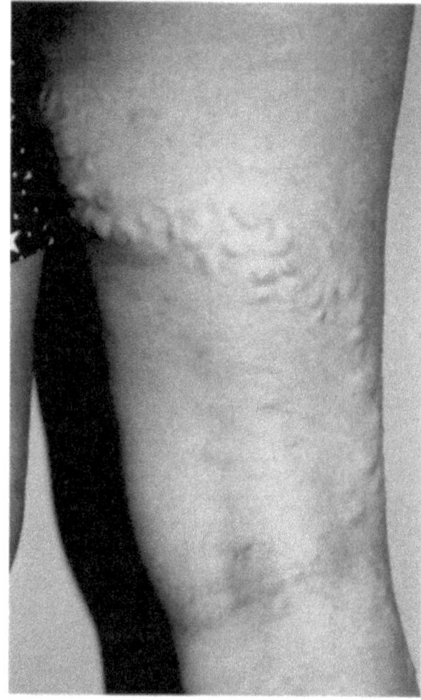

Figure 5.8 This pattern of varicose veins is common. In this case they derived from varicose pudendal veins but they may be caused from an incompetent posterior medial branch of the greater saphenous vein. It is important to follow the vein upward with a Doppler to determine the exact origin of reflux.

A familiar sight to the sclerotherapist is the combination of incompetent lateral thigh veins joined to a sun burst of spidery telangiectasias on the upper thigh. This type of venous disorder responds well to injection sclerotherapy as shown in Plate 2.

Principles of treating varicose veins

If we are to expect the best results when treating varicose veins certain basic principles should be fulfilled.

Allow etiologic factors to subside

Although most varicose veins take many years to develop there are some which are precipitated or aggravated by recent events.

Pregnancy

When primary varicose veins develop during pregnancy most phlebologists wait 1–2 months after delivery or after the cessation of breast feeding to begin treatment. This allows hormonal influences to abate and the body's blood volume, retained water and extra weight to normalize.

In the past many physicians recommended that women with pregnancy-related varices should wait until they had completed their families before having their veins treated. The idea was that the stripping operation was so unpleasant that no woman would want the procedure repeated after further pregnancies.

Most of us now believe that varicose disease should be treated after any pregnancy regardless of future plans for more children. Treating current disease helps to protect normal veins from the devastating effects of future pregnancies. Current treatment options are less traumatic than was formerly the case.

Acute superficial phlebitis

Phlebitis may be the presenting event which sends the patient to the doctor for treatment of chronic varicose disease. Other than compression, treatment should be delayed for a number of months or until the inflammation and swelling are completely resolved. Adequate compression during the acute stage of the phlebitis will often cause the involved veins to sclerose, closing them as if they have been treated with sclerotherapy.

Deep venous thrombosis

When varicose veins develop secondary to DVT they too should not be treated until the acute process has resolved. Some phlebologists wait a year after a DVT to treat secondary varices. On the other hand the secondary varices often do not develop for a long time after the initial process. Veins which have been involved with a phlebitic process are often more fragile and susceptible to sclerosants than normal varicose veins. Treatment may initiate further thrombophlebitis if undertaken too soon.

Demonstrate deep venous outflow patency

For surface varicose veins to be treated it must first be shown that they are not a collateral or bypass for a deep venous obstruction. This fact has been addressed and may require ultrasonography, plethysmography or venographic methods to verify an adequate outflow tract when there has been a previous DVT. When purely superficial incompetence is shown there is no problem in initiating treatment. [2]

Obliterate proximal points of reflux

A major premise in contemporary phlebology is that appropriate treatment must, if at all possible, obliterate the most proximal points of reflux. The French call this "the leak"; they say for example that when it rains there will always be water in the basement as long as there is a leak in the roof.

From a clinical standpoint we know that if only visible varicose veins are treated, and an incompetent saphenous junction or perforator goes unnoticed, the likelihood of new varicose veins developing markedly increases. This premise emphasizes the need for accurate pre-treatment testing to determine the highest or most proximal point of reflux.

In the case of large varicose veins which originate from one of the saphenous veins the "leak" is at the saphenous junctions with the deep vein or from incompetent perforating veins. The saphenous trunk becomes the conduit which transmits the hydrostatic pressure. The varicose vein is the end point of the venous insufficiency.

In many cases where the saphenous trunks were once incompetent but regained competence (e.g. pregnancy) the highest point of reflux is at the origin of the varicose tributary itself. Pre-treatment testing determines whether the saphenous trunks are competent and the source of reflux.

In the case of vulval or pudendal veins the source of reflux is within the pelvis. It may not be possible to meet the principle of obliterating the highest point of reflux unless the pelvic veins are obliterated. For this reason the patient must be cautioned that new varicosities may develop and repeat treatment may be necessary.

Treat from proximal to distal

This principle follows the previous one. Optimal treatment results are obtained when the pressure within the varicose vein is the least. It is obvious that hydrostatic pressure is least at the origin of reflux and increases as the length of the involved vein increases and may not be relieved with exercise.

The concept of proximal to distal treatment has been emphasized by French phlebologists who treat many of the varicose conditions entirely with sclerotherapy. Here a segmental approach is undertaken. The proximal leak is first sclerosed breaking the reflux cycle. The distal segment is allowed to shrink and then treated. Each treated segment lowers the pressure of the segment below. The varicose system is successively treated until all elements are obliterated.

Fegan's original treatment method relied on total sclerotherapy as well, yet differed in two ways. First it appeared to be contrary to the principle of starting at the top and working down. The technique does in fact start the injections at the bottom of the leg and works upward; however, the entire leg is sclerosed in one session. His technique emphasizes the need of finding and injecting incompetent perforating veins, which in this method are the "leaks".

In the USA, surgical treatment has been the traditional method of eradicating varicose veins. In past years the saphenous vein was always stripped. This approach eliminated any possible source of reflux along the course of the saphenous vein. Of course parts or all of the vein may have been normal.

Contemporary treatment methods use both the segmental and total treatment methods. If the leak is at the saphenofemoral or SPJ this is always a site of treatment. A single session approach might involve clipping the SFJ and phlebectomizing the varices under local anesthesia. Alternatively, the junction might be ligated, divided and segmental saphenous vein stripping performed. After waiting a few weeks for shrinkage the varicosities would then be phlebectomized or sclerosed.

Surgeons prefer to obliterate the saphenous junctions surgically because the results are immediate, 100% effective and probably longer lasting than sclerotherapy. Nevertheless many experienced sclerotherapists report satisfactory results with injections placed into the saphenous veins to correct reflux.

Whatever the problem, it is imperative that pre-treatment evaluation determines the source and extent of reflux so that a rational and individualized treatment program can be developed. Adequate treatment demands that all parts of the varicose system, hidden and visible, be given appropriate treatment.

GSV incompetence

According to the principles of treatment reflux in the GSV must first be corrected before side branch varicosis can be treated. The surgical choices are obliteration of reflux at the SFJ by high ligation or by removal of the GSV. Associated larger varicose veins can then be removed by the microincisional phlebectomy hook technique or treated later with sclerotherapy.

There are many sclerotherapists who attempt to close the incompetent saphenous vein with injections. There is little agreement among them regarding long term results or the best method of performing the treatments. [3]

GSV preservation

There is a sizeable group of surgical phlebologists who preserve the GSV by performing a high ligation of the incompetent SFJ. The technique is similar to that used in the early years of the century.

GSV stripping

Stripping is a process by which a long segment of saphenous vein is removed from beneath the skin surface using a stripper wire or cable. Most general surgeons in the USA are trained in the traditional Mayo–Kelly stripping from ankle to groin. Other methods and instruments are described more fully in Chap. 7.

LSV incompetence

There is not so much controversy regarding treatment of the LSV. Most surgeons continue to strip the LSV, a process which should have few side-effects.

Unlike the traditional stripping method wherein the stripper was introduced at the ankle and advanced upward to strip the vein, current techniques are similar to those used for the GSV, i.e. the vein is approached through a small transverse incision at the flexion crease of the knee; it is then isolated, dissected upward to the SPJ and clipped flush with the popliteal vein. The lower section is stripped to a spot below the last varicose side branch. Associated varicosities are treated by phlebectomy or sclerotherapy.

However, the functional qualities of the LSV are different from those of the GSV. For example there are no perforating veins except the vein at the gastrocnemius point. For this reason many surgeons do not strip the vein but perform a high ligation and local excision of the vein.

Microincisional phlebectomy

This technique removes varicose veins through tiny skin incisions. The Mayo brothers proved the effectiveness of removing the varicose veins surgically. But for some unknown reason American surgeons have thought that large incisions are required to adequately expose and excise the varices. This reasoning and its attendant scars caused traditional phlebectomy to fall into disfavor with the American consumer.

Our European and British counterparts have developed a more esthetic approach; a series of 1–2 mm incisions are made along the course of the varicose vein. Because the incisions are so small the veins cannot be seen and are dissected out with specially designed hooks and then avulsed from beneath the skin surface. With patience and care the entire varicose complex can be removed. The technique is useful for most varices of GSV or LSV origin. [4]

Comments

Contemporary surgical treatments appear to be more complete, less traumatic and cause less scarring and disability than those of the past. These findings should encourage physicians to offer surgical treatment to their patients at an earlier stage in their disease.

Injection sclerotherapy now holds its proper place in the treatment of varicose veins. However, there is still a large amount of data to be obtained before we can know whether all patients should receive stripping for GSV insufficiency or whether venous interruption is adequate treatment for some. We also need to know whether sclerotherapy can be used as an effective treatment method for obliterating SFJ reflux.

References

1. Tretbar LL (1989) The origin of reflux in incompetent blue reticular/telangiectasia veins. In Phlebologie '89, Davy A, Stemmer R eds. John Libbey/Eurotext, London/Paris

2. Hach W, Hach-Wunderle V (1997) Phlebography and Sonography of the Veins. Springer, Heidelberg

3. Hobbs JT ed (1977) The Treatment of Venous Disorders. JB Lippincott, Philadelphia

4. Goldman MP, Bergan JJ eds (1996) Ambulatory Treatment of Venous Disease. An Illustrative Guide. Mosby, St Louis

CHAPTER 6

History of Medical and Surgical Treatment of Varicose Veins

Among the first to recommend surgical treatment was Hippocrates, earlier than 300 BC. He suggested puncturing the varicosities at multiple points. Since that time, as Mercer points out so succinctly, "Varicosities have been cauterized, twisted, poked, avulsed, ligated, divided and stripped".

Early surgical treatments

Most operations were directed toward excising varicose clusters and ligation of the proximal and distal veins. Because of the continuing problem of infection and thrombosis surgical treatments were usually reserved for those with non-healing ulcerations. Ambroise Paré (Fig. 6.1) for example in the 16th century became famous for his varicose vein treatments after healing the chronic venous ulcer of his captor Lord Vandeville. Paré described his technique: "One usually cuts the varix on the inner part of the thigh, a little above the knee, where a varicose vein is usually found to develop…for the purpose of cutting the channel and making a barrier against the blood and other humours contained with it, which fills any ulcers present in the legs".

Although Paré assumed there were malignant humours in the stagnant blood he was one of the first to propose the concept of creating a barrier to blood flowing down the leg.

During the same century Fabricius, William Harvey's professor in Padua, noted that large varicose veins emptied when the leg was elevated and filled when the leg was dependent. He performed double ligation and division of a varix above an ulcer and "by

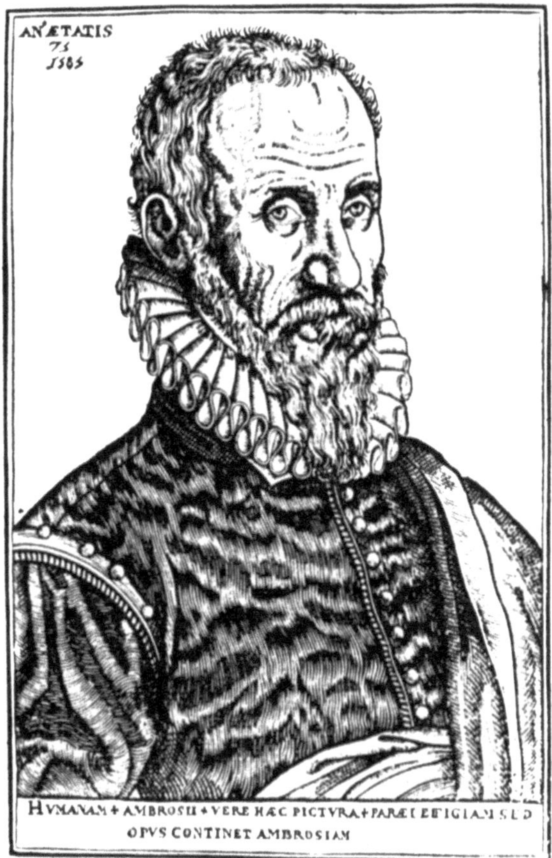

Figure 6.1 Ambroise Paré from *Les oeuvres d'Ambroise Paré*, Rigaus & Obert, Lyon, 1633. He is shown at the age of 75 years (although the illustration is identical to another etching which shows him at 68 years of age). From humble beginnings, without education in Latin or Greek, he rose from a simple barber-surgeon to surgeon for four kings. He wrote extensively and his observations were translated into six languages. Having reintroduced the use of ligatures for war wounds there is little wonder that he should ligate the saphenous vein.

divine favor" obtained a cure of the ulcer. It was not uncommon, as Paré did, to credit "a higher being" with successful healing. If the treatment failed you were exonerated.

British experience

It was not until the 19th century, however, that the real significance of the saphenous trunks was realized. One of the earliest investigators to discuss the importance of gravitational reflux was Mr Benjamin Collins Brodie, a surgeon at St George's Hospital in London. In 1846 he observed that, "If I put on a bandage, and squeezed the blood out of the veins below, and then put my thumb on the vena saphena above, so as to stop the circulation through it, I found, on taking off the bandage, the patient being in the erect posture, that the cluster of veins below filled very slowly, and only from the capillary vessels." [1]

He further observed that, "if the patient being in the erect posture, I removed the pressure from the vein, the valves being of no use, the blood rushed downwards by its own weight, . . . and filled the varicose cluster below almost instantaneously. I can understand that a ligature upon the vena saphena under these circumstances, would in a great degree lessen the inconvenience arising from the distention of the varicose veins below." This was, of course, the famous first report of a test for reflux in the saphenous vein and the conclusion that interrupting the flow by ligature would be of benefit.

It is curious that in the same lecture he mentions that in 1799 Sir Everard Home (the brother-in-law of John Hunter) recommended the application of a ligature to the "vena saphena major when the veins of the leg were varicose". He performed this operation "in a great number of cases, and in a few cases he applied it to the vena saphena minor." Brodie, pictured in Fig. 6.2, tried the procedure himself but gave it up because of severe "venous inflammation" resulting in a number of deaths.

In an earlier communiqué of 1836 Brodie described his original surgical approach. "I made an incision with a scalpel, through the varix and skin over it. I generally employed a narrow, sharp-pointed bistoury, slightly curved, with its cutting edge on the convex side...so that the varicose vessels are completely divided, while the skin over them is preserved entire, with the exception of a moderate puncture, which is necessary for the introduction of the instrument with which the incision of the veins is effected." This sounds like the original description of microincisional phlebectomy.

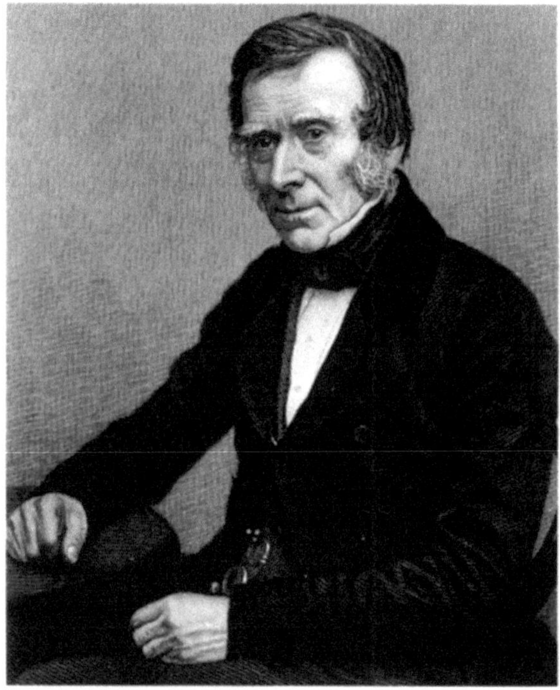

Figure 6.2 Sir Benjamin Collins Brodie, from a photograph by Maull & Polyblank, about 1848. He was then President of the Royal Society, a Fellow of the Royal College of Physicians and prominent in social circles having been knighted by the new Queen Victoria. (Reproduced with the kind permission of the Royal Society of Medicine, London.)

As his career progressed he became disenchanted with surgical treatments because of the sepsis and phlebitis which complicated surgical operations in the pre-Listerian age. He resorted to local treatment and demonstrated the effectiveness of compression bandaging for the healing of venous ulcers.

Brodie was recognized by Queen Victoria with a knighthood, and is said to have reminded his colleagues, "Gentlemen, there is more in veins than just blue blood".

German experience

Other surgeons, recognizing the role played by reflux from the saphenous vein, began to treat it surgically. In 1884 O.W. Madelung of Rostock suggested treating varicose ulcers by excising the GSV through a long incision, as demonstrated in Fig. 6.3. He also recommended "scraping the ulcer bed with a sharp spoon, disinfecting it with zinc chloride and packing it with iodoform gauze". [2] Although a rather horrendous operation, it remained popular for many years, having been reported by Charles Mayo in 1900 as a successful

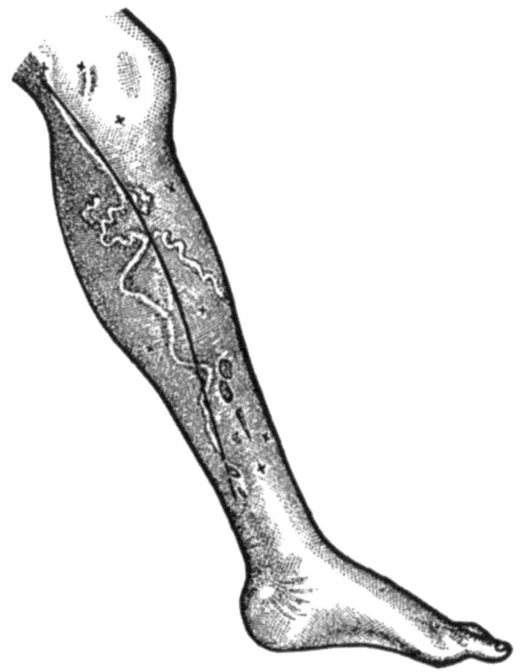

Figure 6.3 O.W. Madelung resurrected the surgical treatment of excising the saphenous vein. His operation probably cured more venous ulcers than other surgical methods of the period since it completely eradicated all sources of venous reflux to the ulcer area. The line of incision along the greater saphenous vein is clearly outlined. Each "*x*" marks the extent of undermining to remove varicose veins. The thin leg suggests that the ulcers were due to superficial venous disease. (Reproduced from the original publication [2].)

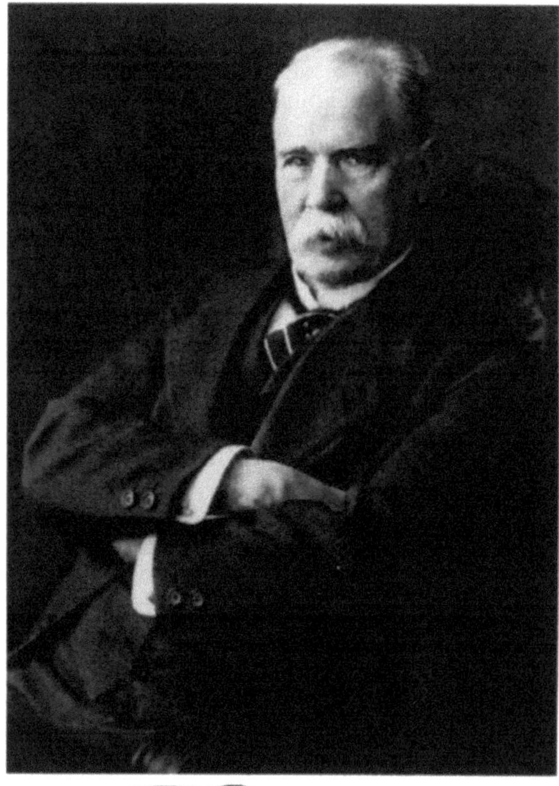

Figure 6.4 Friedrich Trendelenburg in 1912. He dominated vascular surgery in Europe during the late 19th and early 20th century. (Reproduced with the kind permission of the Wellcome Institute Library, London.)

form of treatment. A recent paper reports that the operation was only discontinued in 1988 and replaced by hook avulsion. [3]

When originally introduced it probably was more successful than other treatments because it completely eliminated reflux to the ulcerated areas, debrided the ulcer bed and provided antisepsis.

Friedrich Trendelenburg (Fig. 6.4), professor of surgery at the Bonn Surgical Clinic, in his monumental paper of 1891, re-evaluated the previous attempts at saphenous ligation and concluded, "It was the comparatively great danger of the operation in pre-antiseptic times which brought it no great approbation or imitation. Thus it happened that the true idea was buried in oblivion…" He then described his method of saphenous ligation. "Generally the point at the junction of the lower and middle thirds of the thigh proves to be the most favorable point for finger compression and also for ligation. The vein is exposed through a skin incision about 3 cm long and isolated with the handle of the scalpel. Then a catgut suture is passed around above and below by means of an aneurysm needle…the vein doubly ligated and severed between the ligatures. The operation can be completed

in a few minutes and is not painful enough that anesthesia is always necessary". [4]

Trendelenburg selected the point "at the junction of the lower and middle thirds" where the vein escapes the protection of the deeper fascia and often becomes grossly dilated. He also observed that, "an especially prominent circumscribed varix of about the size of a hazel nut or walnut is usually seen", and noted a similar finding in the groin. We recognize these findings today with prolonged, advanced dilation of the saphenous vein. Trendelenburg suggests the "varix" is caused by the undue pressure exerted in an area usually protected by a normal valve. Actually he describes a "blow-out" just below an incompetent valve as described in Chap. 6.

Trendelenburg's 1891 report is more famous for his description of the maneuver which has become known the world over as the Trendelenburg test: "One lays the patient flat, raises the leg to the perpendicular, lets all the blood flow out of the saphenous field and compresses the trunk of the saphenous with the finger at a spot where it is easily recognizable. Now one lets the patient come down from the table with care, without removing the compressing finger from the saphenous. We see that the whole saphenous vein now remains empty at first on standing. Not until the lapse of a quarter to a half a minute does one see the varicosities in the leg gradually begin to fill with blood again. Only when one removes the compressing finger, does a larger amount of blood rush down from above into the saphenous and the old picture of the tensely distended varicosities returns".

These findings are similar to those reported by Brodie a half century earlier, although no mention is made of his work. This test is now properly called the Brodie–Trendelenburg test and is still useful to demonstrate the presence of incompetent perforating veins, a finding described by Trendelenburg in his original report.

Trendelenburg's disciple Georg Perthes, also of the Bonn Surgical Clinic, reviewed more than 87 operations in 1895. [5] The previous poor results obtained with venous ulcers he believed was because "venous blood low in nutrients flows back into varicose veins". He also recognizes that, "When the ligation is made high up on the trunk there will be fewer side branches above the point of ligation and it will be less likely that one of them will reopen the area of varicose veins..."

Perthes is better known from his description in this paper of the "Perthes test" for outflow obstruction, wherein the leg is wrapped to flatten the varicose veins. The patient is then exercised. If the outflow is patent no symptoms develop. If there is outflow obstruction pain develops in the calves from the congestion.

The results of the combined surgical experience from the Bonn Clinic had a profound influence on world surgery.

Post-Trendelenburg experience

In 1896, Mr William Moore of Melbourne reiterated Trendelenburg's method of testing for reflux and reported his surgical results. In the Liverpool Medico-Chirurgical Journal he says, "Since 1893 I resolved to tie and cut the internal saphena immediately below the saphenous opening, and have operated upon fifteen cases in this manner with perfect results". With trepidation he performed the operations as outpatients using cocaine as the local anesthesia.

The process of obliterating the SFJ, so-called "high ligation", still bears the title of the *Trendelenburg Operation*. It became a standard operation when it became obvious to most surgeons that ligation of the

SFJ was more effective than ligating the vein at a lower point in the thigh.

However, multiple ligations remained a popular approach to the varicose vein problem. The Friedel/Rindfleisch operation created a circumferential incision spiraling around the leg for three or four turns as shown in Fig. 6.5. The incision was carried down to and in some cases through the fascia as the many varicose veins were ligated. The incisions were allowed to heal by second intention. [6] Fortunately this operation gathered little popular response among surgeons.

Nevertheless Schede tried to simplify the procedure by creating a single circumferential cut in the thigh, carrying the cut to the muscular fascia in an attempt to interrupt all of the varicose veins. [7] Although these operations were mentioned as late as 1937 in American surgical texts [8] most surgeons were quick to discard them. Ligation of the GSV rapidly fell into disrepute and the importance of saphenofemoral reflux was forgotten for many years so that local

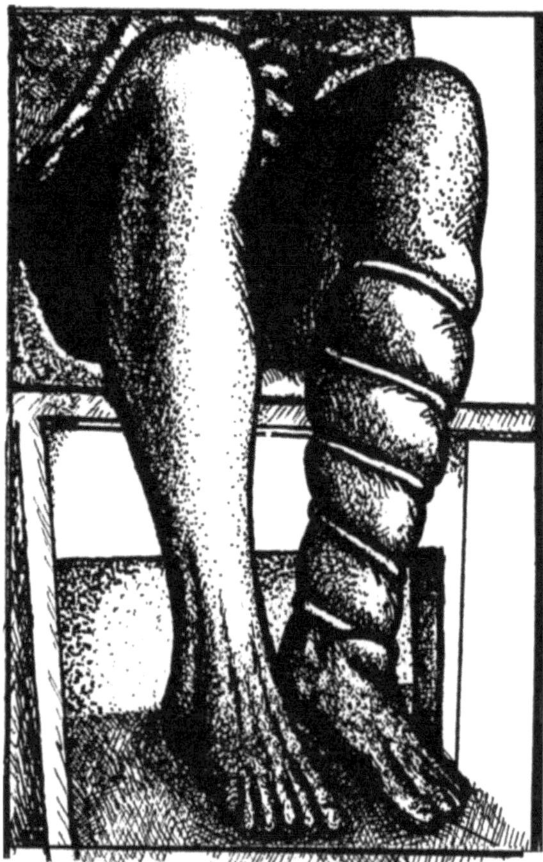

Figure 6.5 Reflux, as the cause of varicose veins, was well recognized after Trendelenburg's proclamation. This operation attempted to treat reflux by dividing all varicose veins in the leg. Fortunately the method failed to gain wide-spread acceptance. (Reproduced with the kind permission of Prof. Dr. med. W. Hach.)

treatment of varicosities again became popular in the early 1900s. Often a combination of local excision combined with injection sclerotherapy was used. But like so many other changes in treatment this approach failed to gather advocates. Usually the sclerosant was too toxic or too caustic, problems that plagued the use of sclerotherapy for the next 50 years.

Improved anesthesia and antisepsis stimulated surgeons to again take charge of varicose vein treatments. Within a few years of each other three American surgeons described new surgical instruments for removing the GSV, a process deferred since Madelung's method of 1884.

American school of surgery

In 1905 D.L. Keller, a surgeon with the public health service in San Francisco, was the first to describe the method of removing the saphenous vein by *inversion*. As shown in Fig. 6.6, a twisted wire was pushed upward through the vein, attached to a suture tied around the end of the vein and the vein intussusepted while pulling it out. [9]

The next year Charles Mayo introduced the concept of *external* stripping. In his 1906 report to the Western Surgical and Gynecological Association he describes a new method of removing the GSV. Two instruments were described: "...we have devised a ring vein-enucleator, which consists of a quarter-inch ring of steel with a long handle, the whole instrument being not unlike a blunt uterine curette bent to an angle near its tip. We have also had made for the same purpose a pair of long forceps, which form a ring at the end when closed".

The end of the vein was threaded through the opening and the stripper pushed up the length of the vein through a series of small incisions. His external stripper and many variations are still in use. [10]

Mayo acknowledged his stripping predecessor by saying, "We have tried the inversion of the veins – Kellar [*sic*] method – but found that ordinary forceps would subcutaneously loosen and torsion out short lengths without much difficulty". Figure 6.7 demonstrates this method of external stripping.

Soon thereafter W.W. Babcock of Philadelphia discussed Mayo's method of external stripping. [11] He stated, "the method is valuable, but fragile, very tortuous or adherent vessels often embarrass the operator". He then tried the Kellar [*sic*] method of invagination stripping but found that "the vein often tears in two before the inversion has proceeded very far..."

Babcock presented his own "special extractor", an

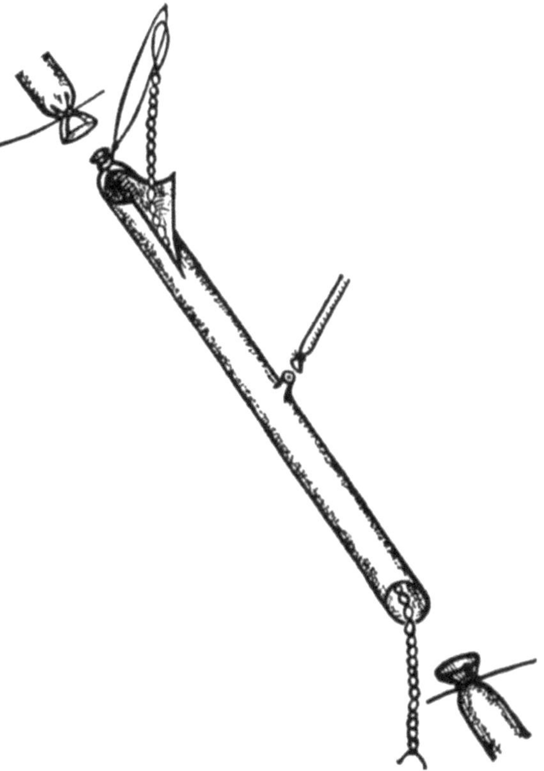

Figure 6.6 With Keller's method of stripping the saphenous vein was exposed just above the knee where it became varicose, the vein was cannulated and the twisted wire pushed up to the saphenofemoral junction. The inversion method of saphenous vein stripping was an original idea which provided another solution to the problem of vein removal. Mayo and Babcock both tried this technique but discarded it because the vein often tore. (Reproduced from the original publication [9].)

internal stripper, 26 inches in length with "bulbous tips", 16 and 24 French in diameter. It was passed downward or upward through the lumen of the vein. A ligature secured the vein beneath the tip: "...traction pulls the vein loose from its surroundings, tears off the venous branches an inch or more from the main trunk, and causes the wall of the vein to be massed or pleated in small compass just below the upper bulbous expansion of the instrument".

With the exception of invagination strippers, today's strippers are identical in design and use to this original instrument. Figure 6.8 shows the Babcock method of stripping with the short, rather rigid stripping device.

The impact that these disclosures had on world surgery is witnessed by the fact that the English words "stripper" and "stripping" are used in all languages. "Babcock" is used to describe the internal stripping operation in many languages.

Nevertheless many American doctors continued to treat the obvious subcutaneous varicose veins with injections. Figure 6.9 is a picture of my father taken in 1910 when he had just graduated from medical

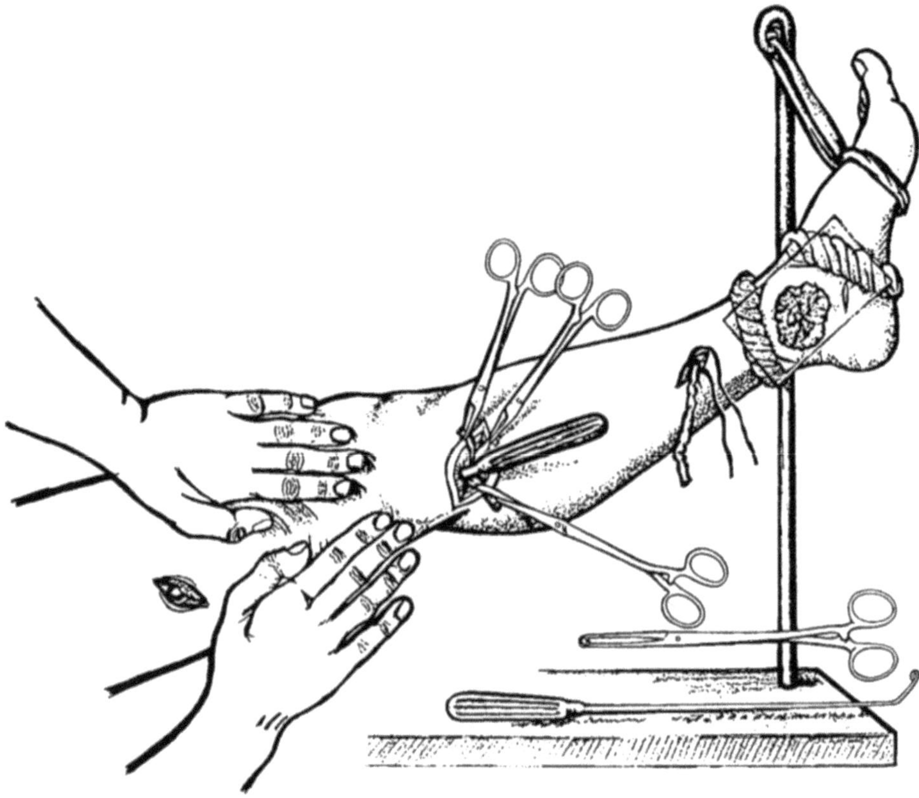

Figure 6.7 This famous diagram startled the surgical world by providing another method of removing an incompetent saphenous vein. An ankle ulcer is covered with a protective bandage during the operation. The saphenous vein has been exposed at various points and subjected to the external stripper. Although the technique gained little international acceptance the surgical instruments were simple and inexpensive and are still found around the world. (Reproduced from the original publication [10].)

school. He not only delivered babies at home and performed appendectomies on the kitchen table but also injected varicose veins.

Later American experience

For the next 50 years every conceivable combination of surgery and injection sclerotherapy has been described in vivid detail. Saphenous vein ligation with and without stripping, ligation and division of the SFJ with injection of the distal saphenous vein, ligation of the GSV with excision of varices and injection sclerotherapy of the saphenous vein and its associated varices have all been described.

Although surgical intervention became more popular after the introduction of the stripping devices there was not an immediate improvement in results. One reason for early recurrences with these methods was that the GSV was stripped only from mid thigh to mid calf, where the vein was grossly dilated. The

incompetent saphenous junction remained a source of reflux and recurrent varicosis developed from the untreated tributaries at the junction and upper thigh.

Other factors responsible for the lack of satisfactory surgical results were the stripping devices themselves and the unsophisticated techniques which needed perfecting. The Babcock stripper for example was too short for adequate stripping and the external stripping methods caused unacceptable bleeding.

Again, disappointment with the early results of surgical treatment caused many physicians to treat the visible varices with injections. Although the use of compression bandaging was being used by some sclerotherapists like Faxon, the combined results of most centers were again disappointing. [12]

So the cycle turned again. Interest was again shown in reflux arising from the femoral junction. Trendelenburg testing became more widespread and in many cases demonstrated GSV incompetence when the vein was not palpably dilated.

As the causal relationship between GSV incompetence and varicosis became accepted, the sclerotherapists jumped into the fray. They attempted

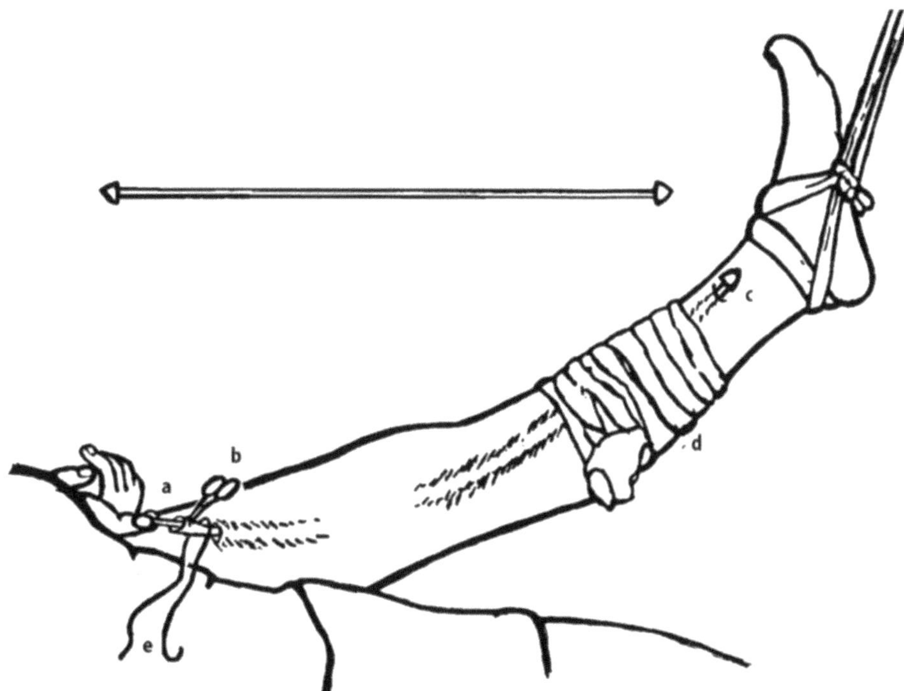

Figure 6.8 Babcock invented yet another surgical device to strip the greater saphenous vein. It was the first intravascular instrument designed to remove the vein by pleating itself beneath the head. The stripper was introduced at the saphenofemoral junction and pushed distally. In this drawing "a" represents the proximal point of introduction with a ligature "e" placed around the vein, "b" is the hemostat holding the vein in place, "d" is a bandage covering an ulcer and "c" the distal point of extraction. (Reproduced from the original publication [11].)

to inject the saphenous vein from knee to thigh. This method too gave disappointing results. Either the saphenous trunk was incompletely sclerosed at the SFJ or it recanalized with early recurrence of varicose veins.

Failure of adequate sclerosis put the surgeons back into the limelight. Homans was an early proponent of high ligation but advocated extensive surgical removal of large varicose veins as well. Many surgeons followed suit and described their own personal methods of ligation.

Most of these surgeons ligated the GSV with heavy catgut sutures before dividing the vein. They also emphasized the importance of a flush ligation with the femoral vein and ligating tributaries which might be a cause of new varicosis in the thigh.

Local anesthesia was used to simplify the operation and avoid the hazards of general anesthesia. Many surgeons emphasized the need to maintain ambulation to avoid the dangers of DVT. A minimal operation under local anesthesia allowed this precept to be followed.

Moszkowicz in 1927 introduced the concept of injecting the distal saphenous vein after ligating and dividing the SFJ, whereupon a small catheter was passed into the distal saphenous vein. Hypertonic glucose was then injected as the catheter was slowly

withdrawn. [13] This approach was quickly accepted by surgeons and became a standard treatment in the USA during the late 1920s and 1930s. Residual varicose veins were injected until they were obliterated. During this period compression of the injected veins was not a standard part of the sclerotherapy treatment.

At the Mayo Clinic local surgical excisions were used until the late 1920s when sclerotherapy again became the dominant treatment method. In 1937 the Moszkowicz technique was adopted. [14] Although the technique of high ligation and retrograde injection of the GSV had been discarded by others it was continued in Rochester until 1947. Their technique is illustrated in Fig. 6.10.

At other centers during the late 1930s surgical treatments were becoming more popular as mixed results of injection treatments were reported. The Oschner Clinic in New Orleans was one of the private medical centers which became involved in the study of varicose disease. Not only did they introduce better clinical methods of evaluating the venous system but they also reported the advantages of surgical treatment, especially when incompetent perforating veins were present.

R.R. Linton of Boston advocated the use of an intraluminal stripper to eradicate the GSV and its branches. However, he is better known for his description of incompetent perforators from the

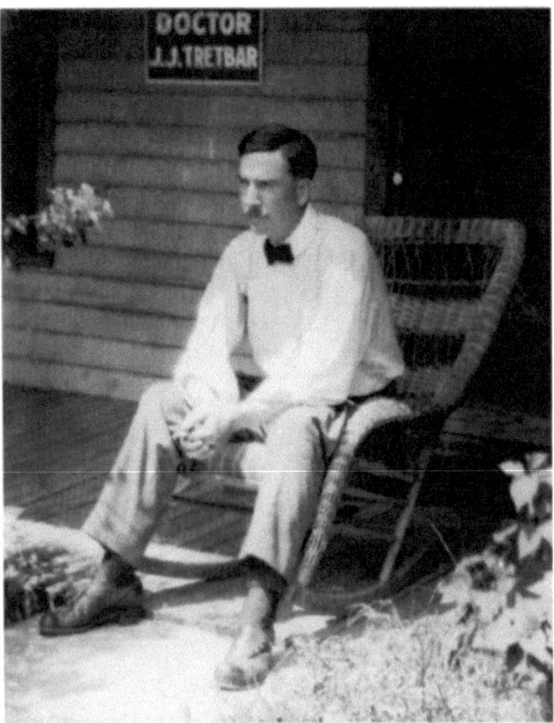

Figure 6.9 This picture of my father, Johann Julius Tretbar, MD (a first-generation German immigrant) was taken after he graduated in the original class from the University of Kansas School of Medicine. The new school was established as a result of the reorganization of medical education following the Flexner report. Upon graduation he moved to a small town of 2000 people, Stafford, Kansas, and bought a small house where he lived and had his general practice. His practice encompassed obstetrics, surgery, pediatrics, internal medicine and injecting varicose veins. His sclerotherapy solution was probably urea.

posterior tibial vein. [15] The "Linton procedure" is still employed occasionally to eradicate incompetent

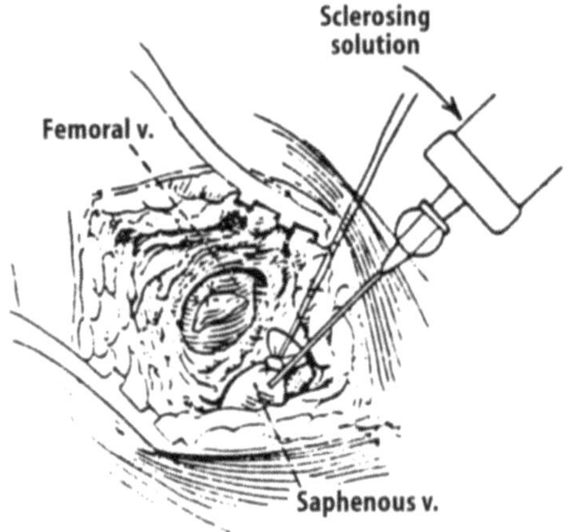

Figure 6.10 This diagram demonstrates the Mayo method of the Moszkowicz operation. In this illustration the saphenous vein has been ligated and cut. A needle is inserted into the distal vein and the sclerosant injected. (Reproduced from the original publication [14].)

perforating veins of the Cockett type. It involves a long incision along the course of the veins on the medial calf, opening the muscular fascia and ligating the perforating veins in the subfascial position. These are the veins thought to be responsible for most of the varicose ulcerations on the medial ankle. A number of variations of this operation have been described and new instruments devised for eradicating the perforators. This approach has been largely discarded as the results are uncertain and poor healing of the liposclerotic tissue is almost universal.

During this period many patients and physicians became disenchanted with the complications of sclerotherapy. Widely used sclerosants were quinine hydrochloride combined with urethane, hypertonic saline and glucose, as was sodium salicylate and sodium morrhuate. Frequent allergic reactions were reported with sodium morrhuate solutions, this sclerosant having been derived from fish oils. A new constitution of sodium morrhuate is now available.

The chemical response of the sclerosants was unpredictable. Either the solution was too weak or too caustic. Rather severe chemical burns occurred along the course of the GSV as well as in the varices themselves. Many failures were reported especially when the GSV itself was injected in an attempt to obliterate it.

Finally in 1947 the Mayo group embarked on a purely surgical approach to the treatment of varicose veins. Their disappointment with previous injection treatments led them to become increasingly aggressive with their surgical treatments. Myers, of the Mayo group, described complete stripping of the saphenous vein from groin to ankle. [16,17] The associated varices were removed as completely as possible through multiple long incisions. The treatment was known as *radical stripping and ligation*. In the hands of the Mayo surgeons a 4–6 h operation was required to eradicate the veins.

The procedures had finally become refined due to better anesthesia and to a number of technical changes in instrumentation. Although the stripper was of the internal Babcock type it was made of flexible cable, developed during the war for aircraft controls.

For the first few years the GSV was stripped only from groin to upper calf and the distal GSV was injected with a sclerosant. However, dissatisfaction with the results of this method caused the surgeons to become more radical with the stripping carried from the ankle to the groin. Residual varices were injected using sodium morrhuate or sodium tetradecyl sulfate. Figure 6.11 illustrates the method of long stripping with the new flexible stripper developed at the Mayo Clinic.

This change of treatment philosophy allowed the Mayo Clinic to compare their own results of high ligation to the stripping method. They found the high

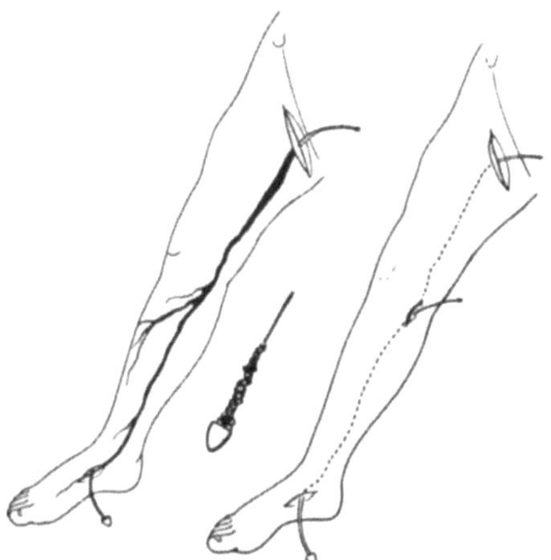

Figure 6.11 The original Babcock instrument has been modified to provide a variety of sizes of stripper heads and cable lengths. The illustration shows how the stripper is passed upward from the ankle. The vein plicates itself below the head as the cable is withdrawn. (Reproduced from the original publication.)

ligation/injection group had only 40% good–excellent results and 55% poor results. The stripping/ligation group reported 94% good–excellent results, no poor results and only 6% fair results. As with most reports of that period the data were often anecdotal and statistical methods were lacking. Yet there is no chance of confusing the overall results. [18]

High recurrence rates in the ligation/injection group (Moszkowicz operation) were attributed to incomplete ligation of the SFJ, recanalization of injected veins and the presence of persistent perforating veins along the injected GSV. It may also be that injection of the GSV injured otherwise competent perforating veins. These perforators, once injured, were rendered incompetent and became the source of new varices.

Review of a subset within the stripping group is also enlightening. One group had intraluminal stripping from groin to knee with injection of the distal GSV. This group showed a 19% recurrence after 2¹/₂ years as compared to a 2% recurrence of the group which had complete stripping from ankle to groin and extensive excision of all varices.

These and similar reports turned American sentiments toward surgery and the popularity of injection sclerotherapy waned with most physicians. The findings made radical stripping and excisions the standard surgical approach in the USA and has remained so until the past few years.

The introduction of stripping into Britain and Europe was welcomed by many surgeons [19], though it fired the controversy which had existed for many years between surgeons and sclerotherapists. One must remember that in the USA and Britain venous disease is treated primarily by the surgeon, whereas in many parts of Europe medical phlebologists and dermatologists assume responsibility.

Finally American surgeons had found a surgical method of eliminating varicose veins with the best long-term results obtained so far. Unfortunately most American women were outraged with the prolonged disability and disfiguring scars which developed from the operation. Scarring as well as the need for a general anesthetic, hospitalization and a painful recovery have given radical surgical treatments a bad reputation in the USA.

In the meantime a resurgence of interest in injection sclerotherapy developed. Tournay in France, Sigg in Switzerland and Fegan in Ireland were reporting improved results utilizing new methods of injection sclerotherapy. [20–22] The principal change in technique was the use of prolonged compression of the injected veins.

Safer and more reliable sclerosant solutions were also introduced. A better understanding of the process of sclerosis, especially the role of compression, improved the efficacy of sclerotherapy. In the USA, Orbach and this author presented early reports showing improved results from compression/sclerotherapy. [23,24]

Not only did the compression/sclerotherapy technique improve long term results, its use for obliterating large truncal varicosities helped to overcome the problem of scarring associated with traditional surgical phlebectomy.

Unfortunately sclerotherapy has not been taught in American medical schools and failed to gain widespread acceptance when introduced from abroad. American surgeons have therefore continued to treat saphenous disease with foot-to-groin stripping and large-incisional phlebectomy.

Follow-up

Many women who develop new varicose veins fail to return for follow up treatment, fearing more disfiguring surgery. Many in fact claim that their varicose veins are worse than they were before operation.

Contemporary evaluation frequently finds a stump of the original saphenous vein with incompetent side branches as the cause of the new varicosis. The residual stump is accompanied with a low groin incision which did not allow complete removal of the vein and its tributaries.

The explanation is simple. We were taught that the SFJ lay three finger-breadths lateral to the pubic symphysis and three finger-breadths below the inguinal ligament, which is correct. Using the traditional method the stripper is introduced at the ankle and advanced upward to the groin. The technique certainly permits an easy passage of the stripper through the valves. Many American surgeons were taught that when the stripper head was felt in the upper thigh a counter-incision was made at that site and the stripper extracted through it. This appeared to be at the proper position, three finger-breadths *below*. Unfortunately it was below the inguinal crease, not the inguinal ligament. This point seldom overlies the actual SFJ but represents the place where the stripper meets the curve of the vein a few cms below the groin crease. This problem is represented diagrammatically in Fig. 6.12.

Recent advances in surgical technique and instrumentation are helping to avoid these problems and are discussed in Chap. 7.

Comments

A historical review of this dimension reminds us that many inventive and resourceful physicians have looked for easier, better or improved treatment methods. Every conceivable combination of treatment methods has been attempted. As the doctors of the past have evaluated their predecessors' work, we too must re-evaluate the current treatment methods, their results and complications.

Today as during the past century we ask the same questions about treatment; should we use sclerotherapy; what is the role of surgery in the treatment of varicose veins; is surgery always necessary to treat large veins; and when necessary just how much surgery is needed? Hopefully we will continue to carefully evaluate our treatment methods and their results.

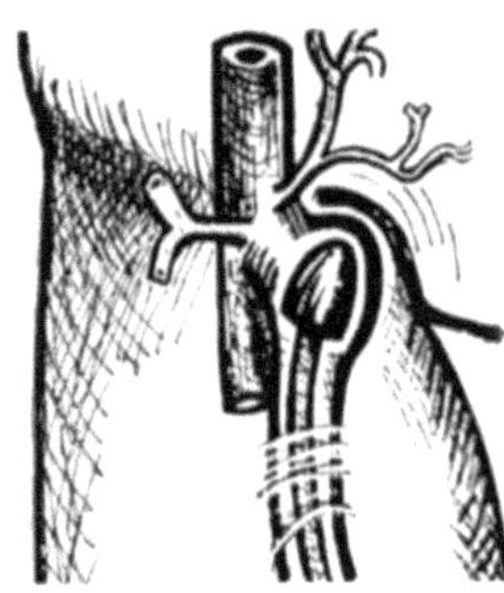

Figure 6.12 This drawing shows how the stripper bumps into the saphenous vein below the actual junction when it is passed from below. If the upper incision is made at this point side branches and a stump may be left behind.

References

1. Brodie BC (1846) Lectures Illustrative of Various Subjects in Pathology and Surgery, Lecture VIII, On Varicose Veins and Ulcers of the Legs. Longmans, London, pp 157–164

2. Madelung OW (1884) Ueber die Ausschalung cirsoider Varicen an den unteren Extremitaten. Verhandl Deutsch Gesellsch Chir 13:114–117

3. Baricza S, Pfeiffer J, Tollas F, Patakyl (1995) Our experiences with different surgical methods in the treatment of acute and chronic illnesses of the leg veins. Phlebology '95 Negus D et al eds, Phlebology, Suppl 1:461–464

4. Trendelenburg F (1891) Ueber die unterbindung der vena saphena magna unterschenkelvaricen. Beitr zur klin chir, sieb band Laupp'schen, Tübingen

5. Perthes G (1895) Ueber die Operation der Unterschenkelvaricen nach Trendelenburg. Deutsch Medicin Wochenschr 16:253–257

6. Friedel G (1908) Operative Behandlung der Varicen, Elephantiasis und Ulcus Cruris. Arch Klin Chir 86:143–159

7. Schede M (1877) Ueber die Operative Behandlung der Unterschenkelvaricen. Berlin Klin Wochenschr Zeit Cbl Chir 31:493–496

8. Horsley JS, Bigger IA eds (1937) Operative Surgery. CV Mosby, St Louis

9. Keller WL (1905) A new method of extirpating the internal saphenous and similar veins in varicose conditions; a preliminary report. NY Philad Med J 82:385

10. Mayo CH (1906) Treatment of varicose veins. Surg Gynecol Obstet 2:385–388

11. Babcock WW (1907) A new operation for the extirpation of varicose veins of the leg. NY Med J 86:153–156

12. Faxon HH (1933) End results in the injection treatment of varicose veins. New Engl J Med 208:357–361

13. Moszkowicz L (1927) Behandlung der Krampfadern mit Zuckerinjektionen kombiniert mit Venenligatur. Zentralbl Chir 54:1732–1736

14. Stalker LK, Heyerdale WK (1940) The technique of combined division, ligation, and injection of the incompetent great saphenous vein. Surg Gynecol Obstet 70:1094–1096

15. Linton RR (1938) The communicating veins of the lower leg and the operative technique for their ligation. Ann Surg 107:582–593

16. Myers TT (1955) Management of varicose veins with special reference to the stripping operation. Surg Clin N Amer 35:1147–1173

17. Myers TT ((1957) Results and technique of stripping operation for varicose veins. JAMA 163:887–892

18. Lofgren KA, Ribisi AP, Myers TT (1958) An evaluation of stripping versus ligation for varicose veins. AMA Arch Surg 76:310–316

19. Rose SS (1993) Historical development of varicose vein surgery. In Varicose Veins and Telangiectasias, Diagnosis and Treatment. Bergan JJ and Goldman MP eds, Quality Medical Publishing, St Louis

20. Tournay R (1966) Traitment sclerosant des tres fines varicosites intra ou sous-dermiques. Soc Fran Phleb 19:235–238

21. Sigg K (1952) The treatment of varicosities and accompanying complications. Angiology 3:355–361

22. Fegan WG (1963) Continuous compression technique of injecting varicose veins. Lancet 2:109–116

23. Orbach EJ (1944) Sclerotherapy of varicose veins: utilization of intravenous air block. Am J Surg 66:362–667

24. Tretbar LL, Pattisson PH (1970) Injection–compression treatment of varicose veins. Am J Surg 120:539–541

CHAPTER 7

Contemporary Medical and Surgical Treatment of Varicose Veins

We have seen in former chapters how every type, variety and combination of treatments have been attempted during the past hundred years or so. With this background of accomplishment and failure it is surprising that any new methods of management might be developed. Nevertheless former surgical operations have been scrutinized, their complications evaluated, their advantages retained and some new methods adopted.

Overview

"Stripping and ligation" is still the standard operation taught to American surgeons. It is usually performed under general anesthesia, the vein removed from ankle to groin and as many of the associated varicosities ligated through incisions large enough to see and grasp the varicose veins. A hospital stay of a few days usually accompanies the operation and bed rest of a few weeks is advised.

Although surgeons have been pleased with good treatment results the American public has not appreciated the disability, the scars and occasional nerve damage. With this unpleasant reputation many people with varicose veins have avoided treatment entirely or have refused to return for treatment when recurring varicose veins develop. In fact many claim that the veins are worse after the surgery than before.

During recent years the British and Europeans have been reviewing their surgical methods and have improved their techniques. In 1962 Dr Jean van der Stricht, a vascular surgeon from Brussels, revived the invagination method of stripping first reported in 1905 by the American surgeon Keller (see Chap. 6). Van der Stricht's reports showed less nerve damage, more rapid ambulation and improved healing during the post operative period. [1] These findings may be due to the fact that the invagination technique does not use the bullet-shaped end of the Babcock stripper which can cause excessive trauma to the subcutaneous tissues and which requires larger incisions for retrieval of the stripper.

Another advance in the stripping technique was to discover that stripping need only be advanced from the groin to the upper calf, where most of the varicose branches occur. Few direct perforating veins are attached to the GSV below the knee. [2] Not only has this approach simplified the operation but it has significantly reduced saphenous nerve injury.

Stripping only to the calf is an anathema to American surgeons who have held to the original findings of the Mayo Clinic experience. The Clinic initially stripped from groin to upper calf but were unhappy with the results so then performed a complete stripping from ankle to groin.

As is often the case, a review of the original technique unearths some useful information. The saphenous veins were stripped from groin to calf whereas the retained distal saphenous was injected with a strong sclerosant. It should be remembered that injection of the upper saphenous vein had been discarded because of the many new varicose veins developing after treatment. I would suggest that the same problem arose by injecting the LSV. It is more than probable that the sclerosant damaged normal perforating veins and that severe varicose veins developed as a result of the treatment itself. Although this is pure conjecture our current results with

LSV preservation can only indict the sclerosant for the poor results observed with the former method of limited stripping.

During this period of improvement with the stripping operation the Swiss and others were developing a new technique of removing larger varicose veins through tiny incisions. Dr Robert Müller, a dermatologist from Neuchatel, is attributed with the development of this revolutionary surgical method. Because surgery had always been performed in a hospital setting and the new phlebectomy technique was performed in the office it was called "ambulatory phlebectomy". [3] As is usually the case other phlebologists were developing similar phlebectomy techniques.

Small skin incisions, 1–2 mm in length, are created over the subcutaneous varicose vein. Because the minuscule incision does not expose the varicose vein to view, a tiny hook or hemostat is used to draw the vein to the surface for removal.

A number of different shapes and sizes of hooks have been developed by various surgeons. Some are blunt and some sharp-ended to meet specific hooking demands. The Müller hooks are more familiar to phlebectomists but were actually devised by Dr Robert Vergereau of Royat, France who named them in honor of his teacher.

The technique is now known by a variety of names. In Europe it is still called "ambulatory phlebectomy", in Australia "nick and pick", by some wags "stab and grab" but usually "stab avulsion". I prefer the more descriptive term "microincisional phlebectomy".

This technique has almost revolutionized the treatment of larger varicose veins. Although the large varicose side branches can be treated with sclerotherapy, phlebectomy can eradicate them more quickly and efficiently with minimal or no scarring. However, the use of hooks in surgery is not a new development as can be seen in Fig. 7.1.

GSV incompetence

Recent changes in attitude have been noted above. Nevertheless new data and a reappraisal of results from traditional treatment methods have fired the ancient controversy concerning the proper treatment of an incompetent GSV. Many traditional surgeons still strip all GSVs from ankle to groin. They would wonder whether leaving the lower segment is a significant change in technique. They also complain that it is difficult to pass the stripper downward against floppy valves.

The real controversy, however, centers around the

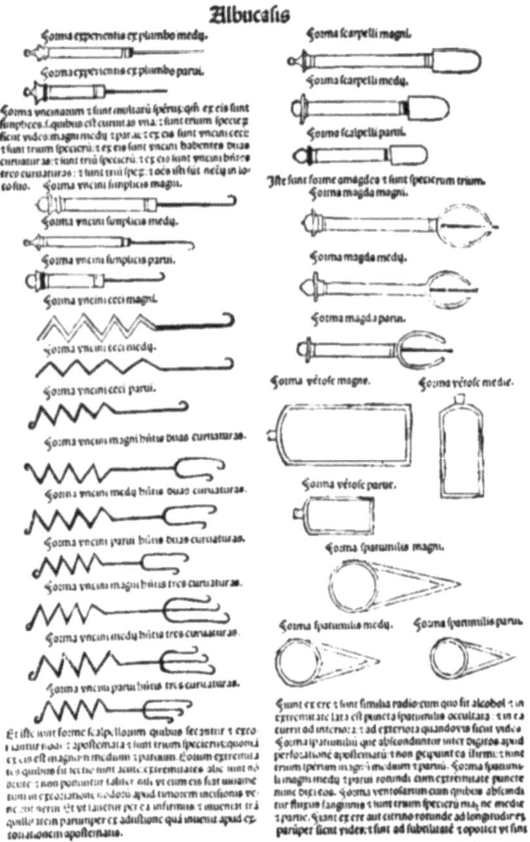

Figure 7.1 This illustration is from a translation of the *Al Tasrif* ('The Method'), originally written in Arabic by Abu'l-Quasim, known in Europe as Albucasis. He was born in 936 near Cordoba and was an extremely influential Arabic surgeon. *Al Tasrif* was an encyclopedia of medical care and represented the first rational, systematic and illustrated treatment on the subject of surgery. It became the foundation for much of the European system of surgery. This illustration shows a variety of hooks, scalpels, trocars and applicators used in his many operations, which included excision of varicose veins.

question of whether it is necessary to strip every incompetent GSV which has caused side branch varicosis or whether there are some which can be preserved. The past history of failures resulting from preservation of the GSV has rightly colored the thinking of most surgical phlebologists.

But when asked the question, "Does every incompetent GSV have to be removed for the best treatment of associated varicose veins?", most surgical phlebologists will say that there are probably some which can be preserved. But when queried as to how those GSVs can be identified there is seldom a consistent answer.

GSV preservation

The following few paragraphs represent the experience of our clinic and the attitudes of the author. The attitudes are still open to revision. During the late 1980s we became disenchanted with the traditional stripping operation but were dubious about the limited invagination stripping method. As a result we set out on a program of total saphenous vein preservation. The 6 year follow-up of more than 500 treated limbs has been detailed elsewhere. [4] Generally anyone with GSV incompetence as evidenced by Doppler reflux of more than 1 s from calf muscle augmentation was entered into the study. The majority of the patients had primary varicose veins unrelated to previous DVT.

Treatment consisted of SFJ obliteration by the use of hemostatic clips placed over the saphenous junction flush with the femoral vein. Some side branches were clipped and divided whereas the saphenous trunk itself was left intact. This procedure was performed as an outpatient under local infiltration anesthesia. Associated side branch varicose veins were obliterated with injection sclerotherapy or removed by phlebectomy.

Follow-up at 3 years showed little difference in the degree of new varicose vein development, about 6–8%, when compared to other groups treated with GSV stripping. After 3–4 years the results began to change, diverging into two groups of generally equal number: those who continued to do well with a minimum of new varicosis, and those who began to develop many new, large varicose veins.

The difference is not surprising perhaps but had not been previously identified. It became apparent that those patients with a SFJ greater than 8–10 mm in diameter, measured 3 cm distal to the femoral vein, did poorly. Those with a smaller starting diameter, 8 mm or less, developed a minimum of new varicoses.

We found that those who did well were usually women with pregnancy-related disease of less than 15 years' duration. The saphenous vein invariably shrank in size and regained some degree of competence. Most SFJs remained continent without reflux. When present, reflux found in the lower GSV came from side branches. In most cases augmentation-induced reflux diminished or disappeared. When present, augmentation-induced reflux often disappeared with exercise, a curious finding. We have reason to believe that the foot pump counteracts low-grade reflux from side branches.

Of the patients showing increased varicosis two subgroups became apparent:

- The SFJ was continent but the GSV did not shrink and significant reflux from side branches caused new varicose veins.
- Marked reflux persisted due to the development of a new, distinct vein growing over the clips from the femoral vein.

It seems likely from the findings of the first group that the saphenous vein has a certain point of elastic rebound. A rubber balloon demonstrates this quality quite well. If you blow it up only a few times it returns to its original size. But after a few more stretches it no longer returns to its shape and remains stretched out.

We see this phenomenon during pregnancy. When the GSV is evaluated, for example during the second trimester, it may distend to 5–6 mm in the low thigh and show rather marked reflux and some varicose veins. Three months after childbirth the saphenous trunk may shrink back to 3–4 mm, lose its reflux but leave small varicose veins behind as a reminder of the pregnancy. Given another pregnancy or two the saphenous vein may not return to normal and remains incompetent.

There were a few exceptions to this general observation concerning the size of the vein. When the varicose condition had been present for more than 15 years, even though the veins were less than 8–10 mm, many did not shrink and continued to grow new varicose veins.

It is our recommendation for those interested in GSV preservation that the two factors be observed: that the diameter be no greater than 8 mm at the time of surgery, and that the duration of disease be considered in the decision.

The second finding, that of new vein generation, is of particular importance. Many surgeons have observed so-called "neogenesis" at the point of high ligation and division. Multiple, small thin-walled veins are often found bridging a previously divided vein. This is not the case here. The new vein measured 4–5 mm in diameter, originated from the femoral vein and ran directly over the clips to join the saphenous just below the point of previous clipping. The vein was thin-walled and contained few if any muscular elements. The lumen was easily outlined with ultrasonography and a probe could be passed through it at surgery. In these cases it required 3–4 years for this new vein to form and the reflux was equal to or greater than before surgery. Removal by stripping was performed in this group and is recommended for veins greater than 8 mm in diameter.

A number of other studies of GSV preservation deserve mention. A well documented study from the UK showed similar results to our own. That is after 3 years one half of the GSVs became competent with few new varicosities developing. The other half continued to reflux and developed a greater number of new varicose veins. Evaluation of the results posed the analogous question of the whether the glass was half empty or half full. The investigators concluded that, because half of the limbs continued to reflux, all incompetent GSVs should be stripped. Unfortunately they did not evaluate the individual characteristics of either group. Of course we must understand that in the National Health Service it is easier and probably less expensive to overtreat half the patients with stripping than to reoperate the other half at a later date. [5]

Critics of GSV preservation declare that almost all studies show thrombosis of the GSV after high ligation. It is therefore surprising to discover that in none of our limbs did the GSV thrombose. All saphenous veins were studied with ultrasonography to determine patency. [6]

Although it is difficult to say with certainty, the surgical technique may make a difference in the matter of thrombosis. All of the studies reporting thrombosis had a traditional ligation and division whereas our GSVs were not divided. It may be that traumatizing the intima by cutting it initiates or encourages thrombosis.

Another common argument for not stripping the GSV is to preserve it for possible coronary artery bypass. Most critics point out rightfully that the GSV is already damaged and not useful as a graft. However, I do not think this argument is germane in determining the best treatment for varicose veins.

One anecdotal case serves as a useful lesson. Eight years ago we performed a SFJ clipping on the incompetent GSV of a 62 year old women. She did well for 3 years with no new varicose veins developing. The same GSV was then used for coronary artery bypass and has continued to perfuse her myocardium for the past 5 years.

Traditional GSV stripping

Stripping is a process by which a long segment of vein is removed from beneath the skin surface with the help of a rigid or flexible stripper. General surgeons in the USA are trained in the traditional Mayo–Kelly stripping from ankle to groin.

Many strippers using a refined Babcock design are still available. The most common is a disposable plastic model which has a semi-rigid "wire" to which different-sized bullet-shaped heads are attached. Traditionally the wire is introduced at the medial malleolus of the ankle, passed upward until its tip is felt in the groin whereupon a counter incision is made (see Chap. 6). The upper incision then allows ligature of the various tributaries (often missed) and removal of the stripper. An appropriate bullet is attached and secured with a suture. Downward traction then avulses the vein from groin to foot. In many cases the bullet actually cuts a tunnel for the extraction of the vein.

As noted the operation was usually performed under a general or spinal anesthesia whose side-effect is vasodilation and subsequent blood loss.

Invagination stripping

Because invagination (inversion) stripping is a relatively unknown surgical technique in the USA it warrants a careful review. Its revival in the 1960s took a few years to catch on, at least in the USA, since surgeons were familiar with and somewhat disenchanted with the Babcock method. In more recent years new surgical instruments have simplified the method and encouraged more surgeons to perform this technique.

Van der Stricht introduced a plastic stripper down the saphenous vein from the transected SFJ and brought it out in the upper calf. A long suture was pulled back up the vein and used for the actual stripping. The thread was tied to the proximal end of the vein, leaving a long tail, and the vein gently pulled out from below. The vein inverted as it was extracted and detached itself from the surrounding tissues.

The long tail is present in case the vein should tear in the process. Then the tail is tied to the distal end of the residual segment and pulled out from above. North Americans then altered the method by using the rigid stripper itself (without a bullet) to invaginate the vein.

A continuing problem occurs when the straight, rigid stripper wire is passed downward. It often catches in a valve sinus or cannot be pushed past a convolution in the vein. To help the surgeon with this problem a number of new strippers have been designed.

One unique design, the "PIN" stripper, stimulated the interest in new instruments. PIN stands for Perforation–INvaginating stripping. [7] It is a thin, semi-rigid wire with an offset head and a perforated tail. The head end is not only steerable, but when passed to the desired distance it perforates the vein, presenting itself beneath the skin surface. Its design allows the inverted vein to be pulled out through a very tiny incision. These features and those of another stripping device are seen in Fig. 7.2.

Benefits of stripping

Numerous studies have demonstrated the merits of stripping the GSV. Unfortunately there are few if any controlled studies which match and compare stripping to high ligation.

Removing the GSV has the advantage of disconnecting it from any of its incompetent perforating veins. It also disconnects side branches and tributaries

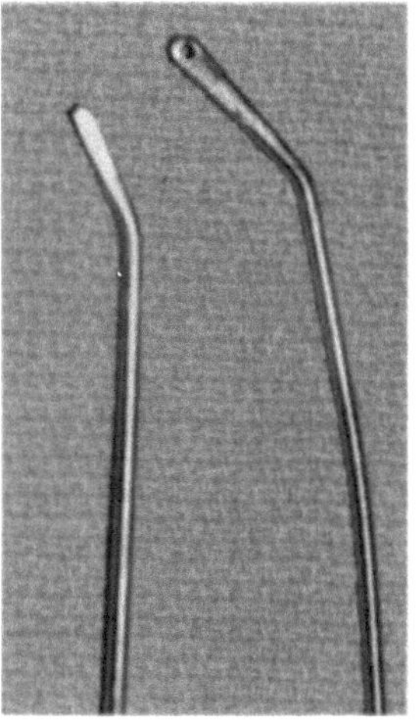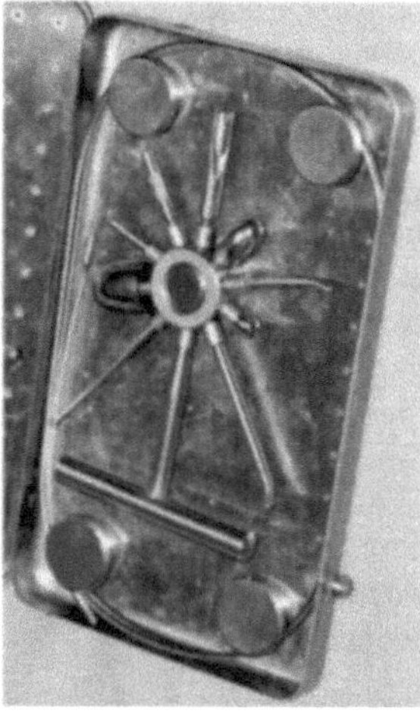

Figure 7.2 On the left are two strippers developed by Andreas Oesch of Berne. The kit on the right was designed by Rheinhard Fischer of St Gallen and offers a variety of heads attachable to a flexible stripping cable.

which can be a source of refluxing blood in the preserved GSV.

In most cases the vein is stripped to the upper or mid calf, usually just past the junction of varicose veins. The lower saphenous is usually competent. There are few perforating veins distal to this point so that further stripping is of little benefit unless there are varicose veins in the lower region.

Stripping only to the calf decreases the likelihood of injuring the adjoining saphenous nerve, an innocuous but disturbing event to the patient.

LSV incompetence

Because the structure and function of the LSV is entirely different from the GSV the treatment need not be so extensive in many cases. For one thing there are no perforating veins along its course with the exception of the perforating vein at the gastrocnemius point. Although I prefer to strip the LSV, a process which should have few side-effects, many surgeons perform a simple high ligation at the SPJ. The sural nerve accompanies the LSV and can be injured by dissection and stripping. There are also small erratic arteries accompanying the veins.

Unlike the original methods wherein the stripper was introduced at the ankle and advanced upward to strip the entire vein, current methods are similar to those used for the GSV: a narrow incision is made at the flexion crease of the knee, the vein identified, dissected to and clipped at the SPJ; the distal segment is stripped using the PIN stripper to the most distal varicose side branch.

Microincisional phlebectomy

The Mayo brothers demonstrated the effectiveness of surgically removing the varicose branches of the saphenous veins. For some unknown reason American surgeons have thought that it required long incisions to adequately excise the varices. This reasoning and its attendant scars caused traditional phlebectomy to fall into disrepute and for injection sclerotherapy to become popular with the American consumer.

Much of the European experience has been with smaller varicosities. Although useful for those in the range of 0.5 cm we still treat many of them with sclerotherapy. Our interest is primarily in the use of phlebectomy for larger varicose veins.

Because the incision is so small the vein cannot be seen. It is fished out with specially designed hooks. The French call all such devices "crochet hooks". A variety of hooks are available, some of which are seen in Fig. 7.3.

To perform phlebectomy a series of incisions are made along the course of the varicose vein, the vein hooked out and avulsed from beneath the skin surface. With patience and care the entire varicose complex can be removed. The technique is useful for most varices whether of GSV or LSV origin.

Secondary varicose veins

Previous chapters have described the process by which superficial varicosities develop following DVT. Continued venous hypertension transmitted from the deep to the superficial system through incompetent perforating veins or saphenous junctions causes the otherwise normal surface veins to dilate. Alternatively the phlebitic process may have progressed into the superficial system, injuring the veins themselves and causing them to become varicose.

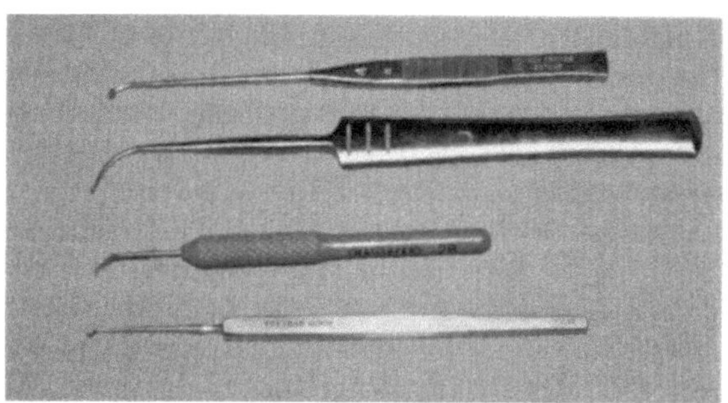

Figure 7.3 This photograph shows a number of hooks which gives the operator a choice for any type or size of vein. From the top are seen the original Müller hook, the Oesch, the Ramelet and the Tretbar hook.

American surgeons categorically refuse to treat them. We have been taught that they represent a potential or current bypass for a local obstruction. Although that may be true during the acute phase of the DVT it is seldom true after a few months or years. Either the obstruction opens up or other large internal collaterals bypass the obstruction.

Nor is it a valid argument to preserve the varicosities, fearing that another obstructing DVT might develop which would require a collateral bypass.

Perthes was concerned about this problem. He compressed the leg and exercised the patient. The absence of pain after exercise implied that there were collateral veins carrying away the venous pool. Pain suggested that the blood could not escape because of outflow obstruction. Wearing compression hose may effect a simple Perthes' test.

Fortunately modern testing techniques can determine whether the offending vein is a bypass or not. Our concern is primarily with the saphenous trunks. Examination shows a GSV or LSV which refluxes with augmentation. The real question is what happens in the vein during exercise. If the vein is acting as a collateral bypass for a deep obstruction the flow in the vein will be upward during exercise.

Our laboratory has been particularly interested in this problem. A number of patients are being seen who have been denied treatment for large varicose veins because of a previous history of DVT. Most of them had only the varicosities with little other evidence of CVI. Others had ulceration, liposclerosis and edema.

It is a simple matter to determine whether or not the saphenous trunk is acting as a bypass.

Valvuloplasty

During the past 10 years a number of surgeons have attempted to repair valves which have been rendered incompetent by vein wall dilation. The early work was undertaken on valves of the deep system, whose function is more important to the health of the leg than those of the superficial system. [8] Unfortunately most of the cases of deep venous smaller insufficiency are caused by DVT where the valves have been damaged beyond repair.

Interest has been expressed in the possibility of repairing the valves at the SFJ. When the SFJ is not dilated beyond 8–10 mm, placing a band of silicon rubber around the junction and narrowing it to 4–6 mm will often restore competency to the valves. We participated in a study using a device which places and calibrates the band at the junction (VenoCuff®). We were amazed to discover that the distal saphenous

vein shrank and valvular function was restored. Blood moved upward through the banded junction in a fairly normal fashion during exercise. [9]

What was equally intriguing was to discover that in the control group, which had only clipping of the SFJ, valvular function was restored in the distal saphenous as it was in the banded group. There was also prograde movement of blood during exercise to the highest thigh perforator. However, when assessed with APG there was no difference in the other parameters of function between the two groups.

Although we were enamored by the ability to restore flow through the SFJ the use of the cuff did not seem worth the expense and time required to apply it properly.

Surgical techniques

Saphenofemoral junction

A rather complete description of the anatomy of the SFJ and appropriate surgical techniques are given here. They are based on more than 1000 dissections performed by the author on patients undergoing treatment of saphenous incompetence.

This detailed explanation is provided because more surgeons with minimal experience are operating in this area and few practical anatomical studies of this region are available to assist the surgeon.

One must remember that this area has many vital structures contained within a small area. Although the SFJ is quite accessible it is nevertheless surrounded by structures which pose potential hazards. Surgical procedures should be undertaken only after one has had special surgical training.

Unlike the junction of the LSV the SFJ is more constant in position, traditionally described as being located 2 cm lateral to the pubic tubercle and 2 cm (or two finger-breadths) below the inguinal ligament.

Unfortunately these anatomical landmarks are not usually apparent in the surgical patient. If the position of the SFJ is to be determined clinically, it is found on the medial edge of a finger placed over the palpable femoral artery. This is in the center of Scarpa's (femoral) triangle, bounded by the adductor muscles medially, the sartorius muscle laterally and the inguinal crease above. This triangle can be seen in most patients by abducting the thigh. Figure 7.4 reviews this anatomy.

In the patient of normal build, the junction is directly beneath the groin crease, the flexion crease of the thigh. In the obese patient it is usually above the crease and below it in the thin patient. Any incision

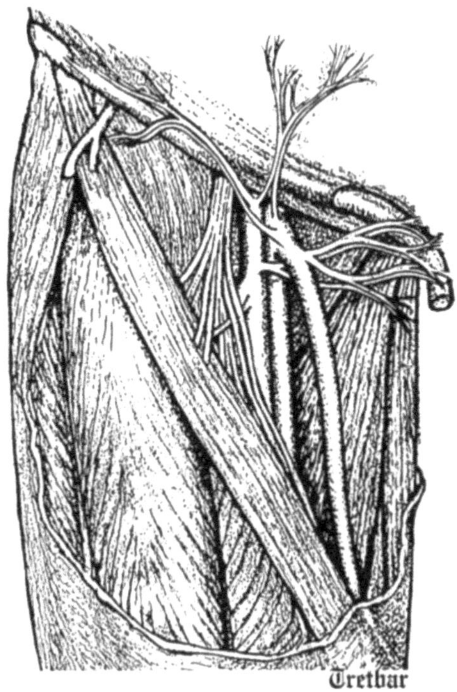

Figure 7.4 Scarpa's triangle is outlined in the diagram. The sartorius muscle forms the lateral border and the adductor muscle the medial border. The inguinal ligament with the spermatic cord lies above the entrance of the femoral vessels into the femoral canal. The greater saphenous vein runs along the border of the sartorius and is joined by the saphenous branch of the femoral nerve. Three major branches at the saphenofemoral junction are joined by small arterial branches at some distance from the junction.

created below the skin crease is too low. A low incision makes it almost impossible effectively to transect the tributaries and ligate the saphenous flush with the femoral vein. Recurrent varicose veins following previous surgery are always associated with incisions placed two finger-breadths too low. At reoperation large unligated tributaries can be found which have pushed their way down the leg to create new varicosities.

The explanation for the low incision by American surgeons has been described in Chap. 6. In this era of portable Dopplers the junction should be precisely identified. The femoral artery is first found and the probe moved slowly toward the mid line until reflux is heard from augmentation of the calf or varices. Its position along the groin crease is heavily marked with a marking pen.

The patient should be positioned as comfortably as possible especially if he is awake. The skin crease can be opened up slightly by abducting the thigh (frog legging). A rolled blanket supports the knee in a flexed position. If stripping or phlebectomy is to be performed this exposes the entire saphenous pathway on the inner leg.

Preparation and draping of the skin must be carefully performed because the medial portion of the skin incision is adjacent to the scrotum or labium. False modesty should not prevent an adequate prepping.

A 3–5 cm skin crease incision is adequate in most cases to dissect the tributaries and isolate the junction. The incision can always be lengthened if necessary. Immediately beneath the skin is typical globular subcutaneous fat. There are no unusual nerves or vessels here. The floor of this layer is Scarpa's fascia. Although a distinct layer, it is quite thin. It is incised and more fatty tissue is encountered – this is more areolar in makeup and can be bluntly dissected. Often a second thin fascial layer is encountered here.

A few fine arterial tributaries may traverse the incision. They are accompanied by an almost invisible nerve which, if electrocoagulated in the conscious patient, may cause him/her extreme reticence about continuation of surgery.

A larger vein, perhaps 1–2 mm in diameter, may appear from the upper portion of the incision and run deeply. This is the inferior epigastric vein and can be followed to the saphenous junction.

If the incision is too far lateral the superficial circumflex iliac vein may be found. It may be running either laterally or in a longitudinal direction. It too can be followed. If the incision is placed too far medially the dissection will proceed down to the fascia of the adductor muscles. Because the muscular fascia is bluish it may be mistaken for the vein.

Proper retraction is essential for satisfactory exposure. Although the procedure can be performed without an assistant, by using self-retaining retractors, this is generally unsatisfactory.

On the skin surface small sharp rake retractors may dissect the upper fatty tissues. Wider blunt toothed rake retractors are helpful as the GSV is approached. They grasp the fat and Scarpa's fascia and draw them apart or tent them upward if necessary.

Small clusters of blood vessels may disturb the approach. They should be ligated or clipped and divided, otherwise they will be torn and bleed.

If lymph nodes lie in the path of the dissection they can usually be retracted upward and the vein found beneath. Retraction is preferred to trying to dissect through the nodes and seldom causes a lymph collection or lymphorrhea. Retraction next to the nodes should be cautious because small vessels which accompany the nodes may be torn.

Lying beneath these superficial structures a blue tint belies the saphenous vein. In most cases it is surrounded with loose areolar tissue, but a dense layer of whitish scar tissue may cover it and hide it from view. Scarring seems to be more common in those patients with a history of chronic venous incompetence.

The actual termination of the GSV is not always

apparent. It may join *en face*, i.e. be an extension of the femoral vein. The two are often of the same diameter so that the junction must be carefully identified. There are no veins joining directly between the saphenous and the femoral vein, so that the two vessels can be separated without fear of bleeding.

Silicone vascular ties can be looped around the distal saphenous. They can be used to manipulate the vein and if bleeding from a proximal tributary occurs they are tightened to stop flow from the distal vein.

The GSV and its tributaries, unless they are grossly varicose, are fairly tough structures. With care they can be grasped and manipulated with atraumatic forceps. When grossly varicose they become stretched and their walls thinned out, making them quite fragile. Here care must be taken to avoid tearing them. If they tear simple pressure will stop the bleeding. However, adequate suction must always be available for this operation.

The tributaries are freed. They join the GSV just at the junction or a few millimeters distal. Of the expected tributaries the inferior epigastric is the most constant in appearance and position. They are tied or clipped with hemostatic clips and divided. Dividing the tributaries initially can help to identify the junction and the femoral vein itself.

The femoral vein is surrounded by a somewhat thicker layer of tissue than the saphenous. Although this tissue is called the "cribiform fascia" it is not always identifiable as a distinct layer. It is mandatory that the actual junction of the two veins be identified. In the heavy patient it may be difficult to retract the tissue enough to see the upper edge of the saphenous as it joins the femoral. A longer skin incision may be necessary for this exposure. Remember that when the incision is placed in the flexion crease even the longest scar disappears.

This exposure also allows one to find deeper tributaries which enter the femoral vein rather than the saphenous. When present they are lateral or medial so that circumferential dissection of the femoral vein is not necessary.

Only after the junction and the tributaries are completely exposed can the GSV be divided or clipped. As a rule of thumb the author must identify at least one tributary at the junction before doing anything permanent to the saphenous itself. The saphenous may then be divided between clamps. The proximal portion is lifted up so that the actual junction can be delineated and any other investigation for tributaries around the femoral vein performed.

When "high ligation" without stripping is performed many prefer a non-absorbable transfixion suture at the junction with a tie placed distal to it. Some surgeons prefer to excise a 3–5 cm segment of distal vein. They

believe this maneuver will help to insure separation of the two ends of the saphenous vein which will in turn prevent reanastomosis.

The author, when not stripping the GSV, prefers to clip the SFJ in continuity. That is, the occluding clips are placed at the junction to prevent reflux but the vein is not transected.

Theoretical arguments for this approach suggest that the vein's endothelium, damaged by cutting, produces certain trophic substances which stimulate the growth of new veins, a process called vascular neogenesis. When the vein is injured by crushing and cutting it releases these substances to the surrounding tissue. The theory suggests that new varicosities, often found at the site of previous surgery, may be caused by this process.

Clipping occludes the vein with minimal damage to it. When the vein is not transsected, the endothelium of course is not exposed to the adjacent tissue. The theory has yet to be proved. Ongoing studies of this approach may shed some light on the controversy. [4]

Closure of the wound is the surgeon's choice. Usually an absorbable suture closes the deeper tissue and the skin closed with clips or sutures. A compression bandage helps to prevent a colorful bruise.

Invagination stripping of GSV

Once the SFJ has been properly treated a stripping device is introduced into the orifice of the distal GSV. A frequent nuisance is the blow-out at the pre-terminal valve. If the vein is pulled taught the cusps will close and the stripper tip will drop into the sinus. Fortunately the steerable strippers can usually find the lumen and advance themselves. If not the vein may have to be dissected more distally and the stripper inserted below the valve. When this fails the saphenous may have to be found around the knee and the stripper passed upward.

The stripper is advanced as far distally as possible. If it hangs up at a twist or bend in the vein the stripper head can usually be steered around it. If another blow-out is encountered similar maneuvering is required. If the stripper cannot be advanced to the calf it may have to be brought out where it stops. The proximal end is tied to the stripper tip and the vein removed by gentle traction from below. Figure 7.5 shows the introduction of the head and the tying of the tail of a flexible, steerable stripper developed by the author.

If the stripper has been brought out in the thigh it is reintroduced distally and the process repeated.

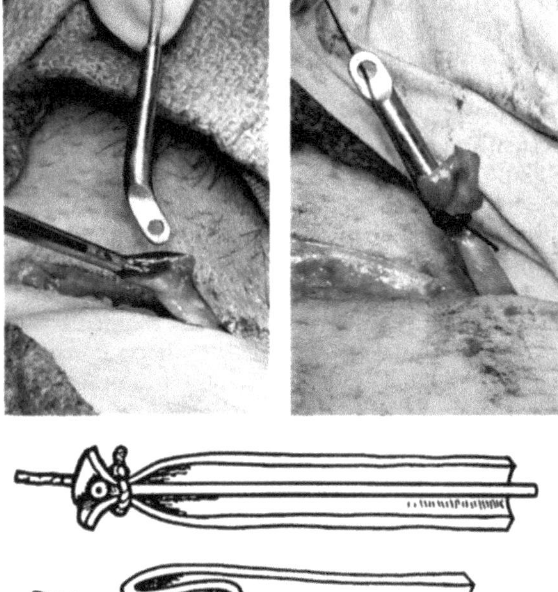

Figure 7.5 The greater saphenous vein has been exposed in the right groin. A flexible stripper head, developed in our clinic, is passed down the vein. The eccentric head permits it to be steered around tortuous bends in the vein. It is brought through a tiny counter-incision, the proximal end is tied and the ligating suture left long. The lower diagrams show how the vein invaginates and the ligature follows. The stripper can be withdrawn should the vein tear during extraction.

Generally we strip the saphenous to a site just distal to the largest cluster of varicose veins. Occasionally the entire length is stripped. It can be helpful to cannulate the vein at the medial malleolus and pass the stripper upward to the calf, as is performed in the traditional method of stripping. The actual invagination can proceed in either direction.

Limited stripping removes the GSV from groin to the calf. This process should disconnect the junctions of the mid and low thigh perforators, Dodd's group, and Boyd's perforator just below the knee. If there are varicose veins originating from the posterior or dorsal arch veins their junctions with the GSV are included in the stripping. This will completely disconnect the varices from any source of reflux.

Rigorous compression is used for hemostasis along the stripping pathway.

Anesthesia for GSV stripping

Although general, spinal or epidural anesthesia is widely used, we and many others have found they are not necessary for successful surgical intervention. Their side-effects are thereby avoided, e.g. spinal headaches, bleeding and nausea.

Local anesthesia in a variety of methods has become popular for stripping. In our own outpatient setting intravenous sedation and analgesia supplement local infiltration anesthesia. A single application, e.g. 1% lidocaine with epinephrine, is injected subdermally next to the varicose veins and along the path of the GSV. Once the stripper is passed and can be palpated, supplemental injections are made directly into its pathway.

The use of epinephrine has had a profound effect on the stripping. Of course it prolongs the anesthetic effect, often long enough for the patient to go home without pain. Its vasoconstrictive effect has markedly reduced the amount of blood loss as well. When using a general anesthesia with the Myer stripper a loss of 100 ml or more was not unusual in the earlier years of my practice. Now 25 ml is considered excessive.

An additional benefit of the epinephrine effect is to shrink the veins. This increases their tensile strength so that they can be pulled with more vigor and less breakage. Being smaller they can also be removed through smaller incisions.

Nerve block of the femoral nerve is reported as a successful method of avoiding general anesthesia. [10] Nerve blocks have few complications except that the block causes muscular paralysis as well as skin anesthesia. A longer recovery may be necessary because the patient may have trouble walking for a few hours.

Another method of anesthesia is the *tumescent* infiltration technique which injects a large volume of dilute local anesthetic agent into the operative area. It was originally used for dermatologic surgery. The technique creates a "tumescence", that is, a bulging of tissues with the large volume of local anesthetic. With this method a larger amount of agent can be injected into a large space without the problem of toxicity.

Invagination stripping of LSV

In most cases the general technique is similar to that used for GSV stripping. The vein is approached through a 3–5 cm transverse incision at the flexion crease of the knee. The vein is isolated and dissected upward to the SPJ. My preference for hemostatic clips allows the incision to be smaller since the jaws of the clipper are quite narrow and can reach upward for a number of centimeters. If the SPJ is higher a higher counter incision may be required. The initial incision allows the vein to be identified in the crevice between the gastrocnemius muscles and to identify any other important fossa structures.

Once the SPJ is obliterated a fine stripper is advanced downward past the entrance of major varicose veins and brought out through another small incision. The vein need only be stripped to this point and not completely to the ankle. Associated large bulky varicosities can be removed by the microincisional phlebectomy technique. This technique is illustrated in Fig. 7.6.

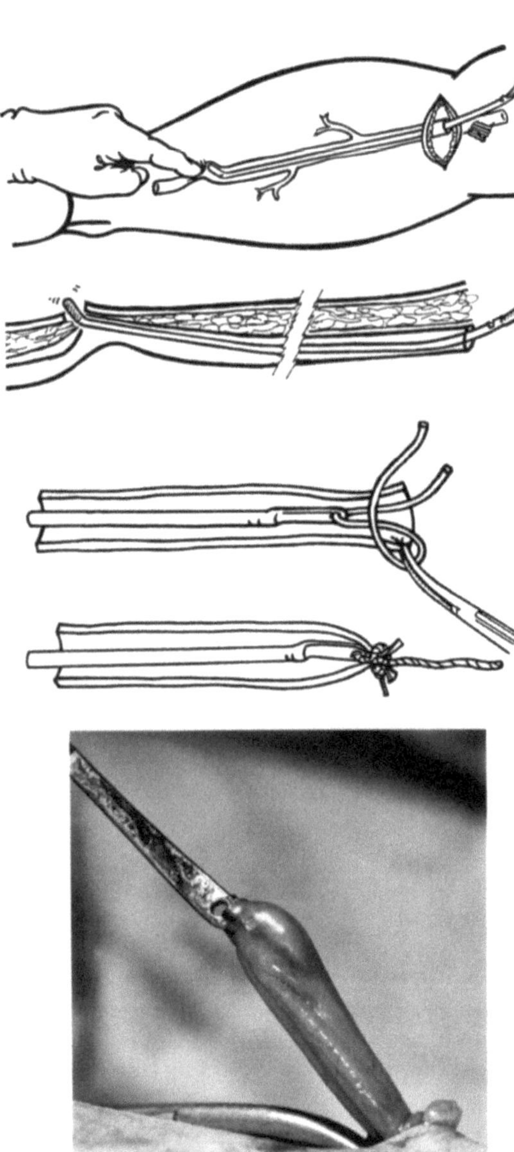

Figure 7.6 This series of drawings shows how the thin perforation–invaginating (PIN) stripper is passed distally where the tip is felt, a counter incision made and the stripper perforates the vein. The stripper is withdrawn, the vein tied on the outside and the vein pulled out via the counter-incision. The photograph shows the stripper and the vein turned inside-out.

Anesthesia for LSV stripping

Because the vein is relatively shallow in its pathway the entire operation can be performed under pure local or tumescent anesthesia without sedation. The patient is positioned on her stomach with the legs slightly flexed.

My preference for anesthetic technique is to use a 30 gauge needle to inject initially a very mild agent at the dermal border, e.g. 0.5% lidocaine without epinephrine. A direct injection into the skin, especially under pressure can be painful. A few moments later, after the original agent has taken effect, a stronger agent containing epinephrine, e.g. 1% lidocaine with epinephrine, is infiltrated into the skin and along the lower path of the vein. It too will require a deeper injection as soon as it is identified by the stripper. Many clinicians buffer the stronger agent with bicarbonate to decrease its painful injection.

The tumescent technique, as described above, uses a larger volume of dilute anesthesia. It is infiltrated into the subcutaneous tissues surrounding the venous structures.

Microincisional phlebectomy

Phlebectomy complements the treatment of truncal varicosis. In most cases the GSV or LSV is the origin of reflux. Most surgeons perform the phlebectomy at the original operation on the saphenous vein. Others prefer to let the varices shrink as much as possible before removing them. Either approach gives satisfactory results.

When the varices are treated at the time of surgery they are marked while the patient stands. Connections with the GSV are especially important and may have been identified by Doppler or duplex scanning. Particular attention is given to the marking of incompetent perforating veins.

The incision or stab wound is performed with a #15C , #11 blade or large gauge needle so that the opening measures 1–3 mm in length. My preference for large varicose veins is the #15C blade which is stubby with a width of 2 mm. It seldom pierces the underlying vein.

One must remember that the use of epinephrine shrinks all of the veins. Tortuous veins may straighten and not appear where they were originally marked.

An appropriate hook is inserted and a search for the vein begins. If one is lucky it will be caught on the first pass of the hook. It is withdrawn as far as possible and grasped with a fine hemostat. A sawing or to-and-fro motion helps to dislodge it from its surrounding tissue. When a loop with the two legs appears it can be separated and each end extracted.

The pulling hemostat must be kept close to the skin surface because the vein begins to stretch and tear at this point. A finger can help break the adhesions to the vein by depressing the skin at a distance from the incision. When the veins are avulsed on either end compression is applied for hemostasis.

Another incision is made proximally or distally and the process continued until as much of the vein is removed as is possible.

A narrow dissecting tool is useful for breaking the adhesions between the varicose vein and the skin. Often the blunt hooks can be used for this purpose.

When hemostasis is obtained the tiny incisions are closed with sterile strips of paper tape. They should be pressed directly over the incision. Traction should not be applied in an attempt to close a gaping opening as one edge will inevitably invert. It is better to place a very fine suture to coapt the edges. Usually the edges gape open because they have been stretched by an instrument used to free adhesions. In this case it is better to enlarge the incision rather than to stretch it.

The leg is compressed and the patient walks from the operating room. The process is tedious but the results are well worth the time and energy required.

There is little post-operative morbidity. Depending on the extent of the surgery most patients return to work and full activities within 3–14 days after treatment. The scars are minimal and usually disappear within a few months. However, some incisions may need longer healing periods. Plate 3 shows scars that required a number of years to disappear. Complications should be few. Ramelet, a skilled Swiss phlebectomist, presents his own experience of complications in an excellent review. [11]

The same general technique is used to remove large varicose veins or saphenous trunks which cannot be stripped because of calcification or scarring. The incisions may have to be slightly longer and more dissection of the adhesions may be required. Figure 7.7 demonstrates this technique. The treatment of a huge, varicose GSV is illustrated in Plates 4 and 5.

Although sclerotherapy and phlebectomy may give equal results below the knee, we have found phlebectomy to be superior in the thigh especially if the leg is large. [12]

With these simplified surgical techniques for eliminating varicose veins and the improved cosmetic results there are few reasons why the average patient would want to avoid treatment of his venous problem.

Complications of venous surgery

Although these surgical approaches seem simple, and usually are, complications can occur even for the most

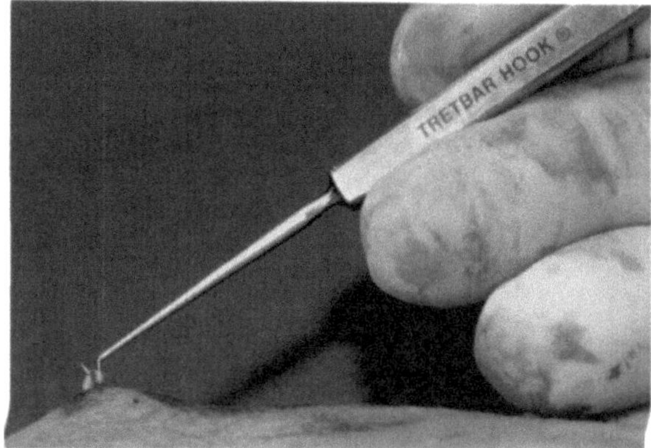

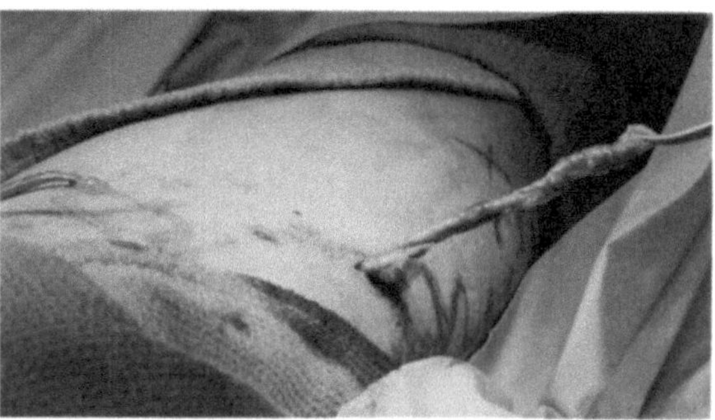

Figure 7.7 A sharp hook is necessary to grasp thicker, scarred veins; dull hooks usually slip off the surface. The vein shown here was 1.8 cm in diameter. It was removed through a 2 mm incision, the vein having shrunk under the influence of the epinephrine in the anesthetic.

experienced surgeon. They may be a result of variations in anatomy, mistaken identification of structures, inappropriate control of bleeding, the physical make-up of the patient and ordinary surgical mishaps.

For example it is quite possible to dissect the femoral vein, mistaking it for the saphenous. If the skin incision is high in a thin person or if the saphenous junction is lower than expected, the GSV and its junction with the femoral vein may lie hidden beneath the lower lip of the incision. The dissection may proceed directly down to the femoral vein which appears to be the saphenous. The femoral vein may be about the same size as a GSV, perhaps 10–14 mm in diameter. However, the femoral vein tends to be somewhat darker and grayer in color and thicker-walled than the saphenous vein. The surrounding tissue is also more dense and adherent.

In more than 400 dissections of the SFJ there has always been at least one tributary at the junction. It is usually the inferior epigastric vein. If this or another tributary is not identified the vein should not be dissected further nor divided until the anatomy is elucidated.

In a couple of cases the author was not sure about the identity of the vessel and clamped the dissected vein with atraumatic vascular clamps and proceeded to other parts of the operation. In one instance the femoral vein was temporarily occluded with the clamp causing the leg to become dusky and dark in color. The patient complained of a tight, strange feeling in the entire leg. It became swollen and the varicose veins became tightly distended.

The clamp was removed and within a few minutes the venous circulation returned to normal. There was no change in arterial circulation. Further dissection showed that the saphenous junction was about 3 cm below the expected level. Fortunately there were no complications from the temporary femoral vein occlusion.

In another case where the patient was obese the isolated vein was thought to be the femoral vein without any tributaries. To identify the junction a stripper wire was passed up the GSV from a truncal varicose vein in the thigh. The dissected vein was in fact the saphenous vein. Further upward dissection revealed the junction with its tributaries.

Obesity always makes for a difficult dissection. The groin crease is usually lower than the junction. The incision should be lengthened and strong retraction used on the proximal flap. It is a better plan to extend the incision than to place the incision higher above the skin crease. A high incision will double the depth of fat to be dissected.

Surgical complications not related to identification of vessels or anatomical variations are equally common. Bleeding is probably the most common problem especially for the less experienced surgeon. Troublesome bleeding is usually related to the tearing of one of the tributaries or the GSV itself or to slippage of the proximal clamp after transsection of the vein. Unless the tear is excessively large the bleeding can be stopped by simple local pressure.

Injuring the tiny pudendal artery, which crosses over the junction in 1–6% of cases, can cause vigorous but momentary bleeding. It too responds to pressure. It is seldom larger than 1 mm in diameter although most anatomy texts show it to be larger than that. Because of its tiny size it may not be identified until it is torn. It should be preserved during the dissection if possible, especially in men. It runs into the pubic area and may help to feed the penile arteries.

The femoral artery is too far away, 1–2 cm, for direct damage to occur. Nevertheless there are branches which when cut will spurt blood. Pressure should be applied but without trying to grasp into the pool of blood with a hemostat. Although I have not encountered aberrant arterial branches they sometimes exist and could be mistaken for the saphenous vein.

There are no major nerves which could be damaged in this small area. The femoral nerve is located lateral to the artery and its genital branches above the area

of dissection. Tiny cutaneous nerves run with the small subcutaneous arteries but cause no problem if divided with the artery.

Lymphedema is an infrequent problem. Edema is quite uncommon if only ligation and division is performed. More extensive stripping may damage the lymphatic channels which run with the GSV along its path up the leg. Swelling of the lower leg can develop and even local swelling at the thigh or knee where the groups of nodes are located. This type of lymphedema is seen occasionally after the GSV has been removed for coronary artery bypass.

New varicose veins

The concept of recurring varicose veins has always stimulated discussion among phlebologists. Those who think their treatments are perfect believe there are no recurrences, only new disease. Others believe that recurrences demonstrate a disease process that can only be temporarily suppressed, no matter how completely treated at the time. We would suggest that there may be two categories of recurring varicose veins.

True recurrences

In this situation varicose veins appear in sites or areas already treated. It is common to find new varices growing beneath or adjacent to previous surgical scars where veins have been excised. Hobbs [13] makes a strong point that there are no true recurrences, only improperly or inadequately treated veins. My own experience suggests that Hobbs is at least partially correct. In the past many American surgeons merely ligated the varicosities at multiple sites rather than removing them entirely. It is likely that the source of venous hypertension at this treatment site has not been eliminated and that the "recurrent" varicosities are residual veins which have become varicose from untreated feeding veins.

Veins which have been treated with injection sclerotherapy may reopen after their initial closure. These can be categorized as a true recurrence.

New varicose veins

Varicose veins which appear in previously untreated areas I consider to be *new varicosities*, not a recurrence. They represent an expression of the progressive and unrelenting nature of venous diseases. It may be that these vessels (like those recurring at previous treatment sites) were subject to reflux at the time of previous treatment but had not yet developed their varicose form.

The vascular neogenesis theory suggests that new varicose veins develop at the sites of previous treatment because of the release of trophic substances from the injured endothelium of the treated veins. This theory has yet to be proved.

Our current methods of ultrasonographic examination may be able to detect many of these early, incompetent but not yet varicose veins. Because they do not yet bulge the traditional clinical examination does not identify them. Now they may be found with simple Doppler examination and be dealt with appropriately at the time of the original treatment.

Contemporary treatment methods may also decrease recurrences because they tend to treat the varices more completely. The microincisional phlebectomy technique thoroughly removes varices as modern sclerotherapy ablates them.

An evaluation by the author of about 100 patients who had traditional stripping and ligations by other surgeons is enlightening. Evaluation using Doppler and ultrasonography showed the following causes of continued varicose vein disease:

- incomplete stripping of the GSV with residual segments, especially around the knee
- low groin incision with a residual saphenofemoral stump and associated varicose tributaries
- new varices in 6–8% of patients in untreated areas
- varices originating from thigh perforators along the path of a completely stripped GSV

These observations strengthen the experience of many other surgeons who demand that surgical treatment must be carefully planned and thoroughly executed. When operating on the GSV certain principles must be followed:

- the SFJ must be completely visualized though an appropriate groin incision
- all tributaries of the SFJ must be obliterated
- the adjacent femoral vein should be searched for tributaries
- healthy veins should be protected by treating nearby varicose veins

Comments

If we view these venous disorders as an "incurable disease" we will not be disappointed with the treatment results. The viewpoint suggests that there may be recurrences and exacerbations. This also means that careful follow-up is of the utmost importance. But it does not relieve us of the responsibility of evaluating and treating the problem as fully and completely as possible. Certainly the addition of sclerotherapy to the surgeon's armamentarium further ensures follow-up compliance.

References

1. van der Stricht J (1963) Saphenectomie par invagination sur fil. Presse med Paris 21:1081–1084
2. Rivlin S (1975) The surgical cure of primary varicose veins. Br J Surg 62:913–917
3. Müller R (1966) Traitement des varices par phlebectomie ambulatoire. Phlebologie 4:277–279
4. Tretbar LL (1995) Correction of reflux at the saphenofemoral junction by clipping-in-continuity: a 6 year follow up in 476 patients. In Phlebology '95, Negus D et al eds, Phlebology, Suppl 1:373–375
5. McMullen GM, Coleridge Smith PD, Scurr JH (1991) Objective assessment of high ligation without stripping the long saphenous vein. Br J Surg 78:1139–1142
6. Tretbar LL (1995) Comparison of externally banded valvuloplasty to interruption of the saphenofemoral junction by clipping-in-continuity for isolated GSV incompetence. In Phlebology '95, Negus D et al eds, Phlebology Suppl 1:367–369
7. Oesch A (1993) "Pin-stripping": a novel method of atraumatic stripping. Phlebology 8:171–173
8. Kistner RL (1991) Valve repair and segment transposition in primary valvular insufficiency. In Venous Disorders, Bergan JJ, Yao JST eds. WB Saunders, Philadelphia
9. Tretbar LL (1995) Hemodynamic alterations in the greater saphenous vein before and after externally banded valvuloplasty. In Phlebology '95, Negus D et al eds, Phlebology, Suppl 1:370–372
10. Fiutek Z, Twardowska-Saucha K, Czaczka D (1995) The method of anesthetic application in surgical treatment of varicose veins in day surgery. In Phlebology '95, Negus D et al eds, Phlebology, Suppl 1:422–424
11. Ramelet AA (1997) Complications of ambulatory phlebectomy. Dermatol Surg 23:947–954
12. Tretbar LL (1995) A 5-year critical evaluation of microincisional phlebectomy for the treatment of varicose veins larger than 1.5 cm in diameter. Dermatol Surg 21:98–99
13. Hobbs JT ed (1977) The Treatment of Venous Disorders. JB Lippincott, Philadelphia

CHAPTER 8

Injection Sclerotherapy

Sclerotherapy is a method of obliterating varicose and spider veins by injecting an irritating solution into their lumens. The object of the treatment is to close the lumen of the vein so that no blood can flow through it. Tiny veins are completely destroyed by the sclerosant whereas larger veins are sealed off.

As elucidated in previous chapters injection sclerotherapy has been used to treat varicose veins for many years. Unfortunately many of the treatment methods and/or sclerosants gave unsatisfactory results or unacceptable complications. As a result the surgical treatment of varicose veins was preferred to sclerotherapy for many years.

The introduction of new sclerosant solutions in the 1930s and 1940s gave impetus to the non-surgical treatment of varicose veins. Better clinical results were reported with the newer sclerosants but it was not until compression was added to the regimen that optimum results were obtained.

Adding compression to the treatment of large veins significantly improved long-term results as it decreased the discomfort and other side-effects of injections. These changes have permitted sclerotherapy to regain its proper place in the treatment of varicose veins. [1]

Mechanism of action of sclerotherapy

Effective sclerotherapy, whether of large truncal varices or small telangiectasias, demands that the vein's lumen must be obliterated by fibrosis. In the ideal situation injection of the sclerosant initiates a process which denudes the endothelium, exposes the subendothelial structures, organizes thrombus and obliterates the lumen by fibrosis. If the thrombus recanalizes the endothelium regenerates and the treatment fails. The objective is that the exposed medial structure heals together so that endosclerosis closes the vein's lumen. Compressing the injected veins decreases thrombus formation and improves the endosclerotic process.

Types of sclerosant solutions

Detergent solutions

Worldwide the most commonly used sclerosants are detergents. Four solutions are generally available, sodium tetradecyl sulfate, polidocanol, sodium morrhuate and ethanolamine oleate. They are all surfactants and decrease the surface tension along the endothelial surface.

Endothelial damage occurs immediately after contact with the sclerosant. In the clinical situation the solution can be seen racing along the vein with even the smallest injection. The detergent agents have been shown to injure RBCs and WBCs but in the concentration used hemolysis is not a problem. Nor does it appear that hemolysis contributes to thrombosis and vein obliteration. The mechanism appears to be that of direct endothelial damage.

Osmotic solutions

Hyperosmolar solutions cause endothelial damage by a direct osmotic exchange of Na^+ which explodes the endothelial cell. Unlike the detergent agents this effect may take many minutes or perhaps hours to develop. It appears that the degree of damage to the vein wall is proportional to the concentration of the osmotic agent. A number of agents are available for sclerotherapy including various concentrations of hypertonic saline. Hypertonic saline has many suppliers and is available in concentrations of 14.6 and 23.4%. NaCl 10% plus dextrose 25% and Na salicylate 30–40% are used in Canada and in Europe.

Chemical irritants

This category of sclerosant is caustic to the endothelial cell by direct chemical action. It too must injure the vein wall adequately to create a transmural sclerosis. The common agents are polyiodinated iodine 4%–12%, and chromated glycerine 72%.

Complications

Like most destructive treatment modalities which require alteration of an epithelial surface, injection sclerotherapy opens the possibilities of allergic reactions, damage to healthy tissue and scarring. Goldman in his superb book on sclerotherapy has made an exhaustive review of complications, many of which are reported here. [2]

Sodium tetradecyl sulfate (STS)

This sclerosant is one of two which are approved by the Food and Drug Administration (FDA) for the injection of varicose veins. Two fatalities associated with sclerotherapy are reported in the package insert of a STS product. Little information is provided and is so vague that interpretation is impossible.

However, a death has been reported for which the details are known. A test dose of 0.5 ml of 0.5% STS was injected into a leg vein of an otherwise healthy 64 year old woman. Apnea developed immediately and she succumbed from its complications. Blood studies suggested an anaphylactoid reaction.

Another death was thought to be associated with a dose of 5 ml of 3% solution. From my personal experience in England this seems unlikely; the Fegan technique used in the vein clinic injected as much as 10 ml of a 3% solution at a session with no untoward effects. [3]

Goldman found 47 cases of non-fatal allergic reactions in more than 14 000 patient reviews. A collective review suggests the incidence to be about 0.3%.

Most of us have seen mild allergic reactions develop in our patients. This may be represented by small hives in an area away from the injection sites. Periorbital swelling is reported as is the induction of migraine headaches and asthmatic breathing, all of which can be blocked with a simple oral antihistamine. Allergic reactions have been reported to develop within a few minutes to days after treatment, making it difficult to recommend testing or waiting in the doctor's office for a period of time. Certainly a well-equipped emergency kit with resuscitation materials and personnel trained in cardiopulmonary resuscitation is essential for the safety of your patients.

Patients who seem to have had a minor allergic reaction, other than urtication at the injection sites, can take an oral antihistamine before the next treatments. Hemolysis with hematuria is reported with the use of a specially formulated foam. No permanent effects are known.

Polidocanol (POL)

One fatality has been reported with the use of POL. A few allergic reactions similar to those from STS have been reported as well. These ranged from anaphylactoid shock, generalized urticaria, to minor regional urtication. Therefore it would seem that POL and STS have similar safety-to-hazard ratios. However, POL has not had the time-exposure that STS has had; that is to say that STS has been used on many more patients over a longer period of time thus increasing the potential of finding more people who might develop a reaction.

Sodium morrhuate

This is the other solution to be FDA-approved for injection sclerotherapy of varicose veins. It has a history of multiple allergic reactions. This is possibly due to the fact that it is manufactured from fish oil with a large residual of unidentified proteins and fatty acids in the solution. Although the product has been reformulated it is still one of the most allergenic of the sclerosants with a number of serious complications.

Ethanolamine oleate

This product was first used in the 1930s to inject spider veins. After being unavailable for many years it has recently returned with FDA approval for treatment of esophageal varices. Many allergic reactions and side-effects related to the large doses needed for esophageal variceal treatment have been reported. It is not recommended for use on peripheral veins.

Hypertonic saline (HS)

Whereas HS has no actual allergic reactions its use may produce side-effects related to high doses of sodium and RBC hemolysis. Many physicians add heparin or a local anesthetic to HS and may thereby create an allergenic solution. The strongest solution that is widely available is 23.4%. It is used at this strength for larger reticular veins but is often diluted 1:1 or more for spider veins. In our clinical experience it tends to be more painful and produces more side-effects than the other sclerosants.

Hypertonic saline and hypertonic dextrose

This combination of hypertonic substances has no intrinsic allergenic potential although the commercial product Sclerodex has added propylene glycol and phenethyl alcohol. The product is viscous but can be injected through a #30 needle; it is sometimes diluted. Its strength is comparable to HS at 10–12% and is widely used for the treatment of spider veins. It is most popular in Canada where it is produced and is said to cause less pigmentation than when HS is used separately.

Sodium salicylate

This solution is often mixed with other sclerosants especially HS. At a concentration of 30–40% its activity is similar to HS in concentrations of 15–25%. When extravasated it is painful. By mixing it with a non-painful solution this effect is used to signal an extravascular injection.

Chromated glycerine

This is known as "Scleremo" in Europe, where it is one of the most popular sclerosants for the treatment of spider veins. It too is viscous and may need to be diluted for easy use. Dilution with lidocaine helps to decrease its somewhat painful injection. Few untoward side-effects have been reported with its use. However,

patients should be quizzed for previous contact dermatitis with white metal jewelry which often contains chromium. These patients should be skin-tested before use and watched for allergic reactions.

Polyiodinated iodine

Although iodines have been used in the past the newly formulated versions have stabilized the iodine ion. Variglobin and Sclerodine are a combination of sodium and potassium iodides with benzyl alcohol added to the solution. It is available in concentrations of 2, 4, 8 and 12%. The few people with iodide allergies should be screened. Otherwise the sclerosant appears to be safe and effective. It is the most vigorous of the sclerosants because it diffuses through the endothelium and vein wall. It is painful when outside the vein wall and can cause necrosis due to its vigor. It is used for veins larger than 2 mm and is the drug of choice by many who try to sclerose the saphenous vein.

Side-effects

By the term "side-effects" we suggest that the undesirable effects of sclerotherapy are less drastic and more temporary than those designated as complications. In a previous review we pointed out that most undesirable side-effects are dose-related. [4] That is, if the dosage is maintained within an appropriate range few side-effects will be observed. Dosage is related to the concentration of the solution, the total amount injected, the length of the injected vein and the degree of blood dilution. Mechanical factors are important as well, e.g. the size of the syringe, the pressure applied to the plunger and the size of the needle.

Post-injection thrombus

Trapped blood is probably the most common side-effect and a causative factor in the development of post-injection pigmentation. Although post-injection compression helps to decrease blood trapping there is inevitably some clotting in the treated veins. This is especially true in the smaller varicose and larger spider veins. Larger spider veins of the order of 0.8–1 mm are particularly prone to blood trapping.

As the trapped blood becomes evident the vein becomes black, raised and tender. After about 2 weeks the blood liquefies and can be evacuated. A #20–23 gauge needle is usually large enough to prick the vein. Gentle pressure expresses the blood. If it does not come out completely it can be re-evacuated at a later visit. The process can be repeated even after a number of months especially in larger veins where liquefaction is slower.

The author's favorite method of evacuating spider vein thromboses is to use a normal saline-filled syringe and a #30 gauge needle. The needle repeatedly pricks the length of the vein as it irrigates the residual blood. This empties the trapped blood more completely than manual expression and is quite painless.

When the blood in a larger vein is thick a larger puncture may be required. For this an #18 needle is useful or incision with the tip of a #11 scalpel blade. The procedure may need some local anesthesia especially when more than one puncture is required.

A few weeks after treatment some patients report an abrupt, painful distention of the vein. Apparently the osmotic pressure of the liquefying blood pulls other fluid into the vein and causes the distention. Pain relief is immediate once the pressure of the old blood is relieved. Temporary compression of larger veins helps prevent the reaccumulation of fluid in the empty vein. Blood seldom reaccumulates since the ends of the vein are already sealed.

Post-injection hyperpigmentation (HP)

This is a common and disturbing side-effect of injection sclerotherapy. It is reported to develop in 1–30% of all patients treated with injection sclerotherapy. HP is thought to represent a post-inflammatory response wherein some of the pigments from the heme molecule are sequestered in the obliterated vein wall or extravasate into the dermis.

Multiple biopsies have confirmed the presence of hemosiderin. On occasion there may be a deposition of melanin in the treated areas as well.

HP can develop after the use of any sclerosant. Even the most experienced phlebologist using the ideal sclerosant on the ideal patient may find HP occurring at some injection sites. Although this viewpoint suggests that HP is inevitable in some patients, there are some factors which may affect the development of HP. Examination of various reports suggests that the percentage of patients developing hyperpigmentation depends on the size and thickness of vein treated, the type and concentration of sclerosant used, aftercare of the injected leg and to some degree the type of skin. Some believe that sun exposure after sclerotherapy can increase the degree of HP although theoretically it should not if the pigment is hemosiderin.

Prevention of hyperpigmentation

The most important consideration in the prevention of hyperpigmentation is to release any trapped blood. Proper compression, by decreasing the amount of blood trapping in the treated vein, is the first important factor in preventing HP. Compression appears to decrease HP in both larger varicose veins as well as telangiectasias. However, the preponderance of spider veins which tend to pigment are on the thigh, an anatomical site notoriously difficult to compress. The early discoloration with pigment is shown clearly in Plate 6.

Injection of a solution too strong for the vein may stimulate pigmentation by burning the vein wall and allowing the release of RBCs into the perivascular tissues. This was true of my original series of telangiectasias treated with a 1% solution of STS. In this group HP was present in perhaps 20–30% of all spider veins and lasted for at least 6–8 months. Diluting the solution to 0.2–0.3% has virtually eliminated HP except where blood trapping occurs. When present the HP is lighter in color and disappears more quickly.

There are a few patients wherein HP develops in almost all of the treated telangiectasias. The pigment is dark brown and lasts for many months. The ankle and foot are prone to this change. In this group there may be no risk factors evident and all attempts at prevention are of little benefit. I have seen only a few which did not resolve within 2–3 years. It is my impression that the "universal pigment reaction" occurs more frequently in darker-skinned people, in lighter-skinned or red-headed people and in older thin-skinned people.

Hyperpigmentation seldom develops in reticular veins 2–3 mm in diameter. They may turn gray and darkish for a few weeks but the brown pigment is absent.

However, when a strong solution is required to close a larger vein, dimpling and a dark pigmentation of the skin are frequent and unpleasant side-effects. This is associated with a localized "perivenitis" and fat necrosis. These findings suggest that the solution used was too strong, because the desired inflammatory reaction should be restricted to the vein wall.

Treatment of hyperpigmentation

Many treatments have been attempted to rid the skin of the pigment or hasten its disappearance. Chemical peels have been used with some benefit. This is not recommended except by those experienced with this technique.

I have scraped off pigmented spots with a knife

blade using a local anesthetic with no residual scarring. However, in a number of patients where I left some pigmented spots untreated I could see no difference between the treated and the untreated areas after 6 months. The pigment faded spontaneously.

Dermabrasion was particularly helpful in a patient who had very dark pigment which persisted for 18 months. The pigment developed as a halo around a deep post-injection ulceration. An adjacent untreated halo did not disappear after another year of waiting and was successfully abraded. This ulceration developed in the early days when a 1% STS solution was used for spider vein sclerosis.

In general no treatment is the best treatment. Although it is difficult for patients to wait, most experienced phlebologists believe this is the best advice. Any attempted treatment risks side-effects.

If the HP is the result of an otherwise judicious treatment it should fade within a year; some pigmentation may require longer. It is also important to take comparative photographs so that the patient can be convinced of the improvement. Although we do not recommend tanning, most patients find that a slight tan hides much of the discoloration. Because the pigment is hemosiderin it should not darken with ultraviolet exposure. For the same reason it should not respond to any of the dermatologic bleaching agents.

Ulceration

Traditionally it is said that ulceration occurs because of an extravascular injection or extravasation of the drug from the injection site. This generalization is simply not true. The fable grew out of the use of hypertonic saline and of course may very well be correct for this sclerosant.

In many cases there is no obvious reason. That is, an ulcer may form in a patient who has had prior successful treatments using the same solution of the same concentration in the same type of veins. The patient shown in Plate 7 represents this problem.

Nevertheless there are probably some genuine factors responsible for some ulcerations. Ulcers have been reported following the use of all of the sclerosants used at varying strengths. Personal experience and various anecdotal conversations suggest that the typical ulcer develops slowly from 7 to 14 days after the injection. Usually the ulceration develops at the site of injection of a small spider vein around the knee or ankle.

Except for perhaps greater pain than expected the injection is "normal". There is no evidence of extravasation or extravascular injection. Immediately after injection an area of skin about 1 cm in diameter blanches and becomes pearly white. Once the blanch has subsided the area remains hyperemic and violaceous.

The ulcer is usually small, about 1–1.5 cm in diameter although ulcerations up to 10 cm are reported. A central core of necrotic tissue develops surrounded by a ridge of painfully inflamed skin. It is usually treated with antibiotics although it is not frankly infected. A scab forms over the eschar. The area remains painful during the healing process which may take 6–8 weeks. Scarring is variable.

Some factors which we believe influence the development of ulceration are discussed in the following paragraphs.

Dosage

Personal experience shows that dosage is important. When there was no worldwide experience with the treatment of telangiectasias we used a 1% solution of STS for spider veins. Tiny ulcers at the site of injection developed in 10–30% of the patients. Although these were not the deep painful type of ulcers they nevertheless disappeared when a 0.3% solution was introduced. In a similar fashion when one attempts to inject too much solution so as to run up the length of a vein, an ulcer may form at the injection site where the final effective concentration of sclerosant may be 10 times the original strength.

Anecdotal reports describe full-thickness skin loss with hypertonic saline. In one case the physician ordinarily used normal saline to flood an area when extravasation was suspected. Hypertonic saline was inadvertently used to irrigate the site and resulted in the formation of a large deep ulcer. The patients shown in color Plate 8, treated by other physicians, demonstrate the potential tissue toxicity of the sclerosants.

Injection pressure

Excessive injection pressure may rupture the vein and allow the fluid to extravasate into the surrounding tissues. This applies particularly to tiny veins where the resistance to injection is quite high. In this case extravasation by rupture may be the cause of ulceration.

Extravasation

As we have indicated the extravasation theory of ulceration remains a popular concept. My personal experience, together with that of many others, is that simple extravasation at the injection site does not cause ulceration. Daily clinical observations show that leakage or extravasation of fluid back around the needle during an otherwise successful intravenous injection seldom if ever causes an ulcer.

Leakage is seen as a bleb expanding in the dermis and the injection is quickly terminated.

Arteriolar injection

The most likely cause of a large or full thickness ulceration would be a venous injection which ran back into an arteriole. The typical deep ulcer follows an otherwise uneventful injection except that the injected area blanches and remains porcelain white for more than a minute. This sequence suggests arteriolar spasm. When the venous telangiectasia is injected the flow of sclerosant proceeds to smaller and more superficial venules and then possibly across the capillary loop to an arteriole. The resulting ischemia in the area supplied by a small artery would lead to necrosis. The depth and size of the ulceration would depend on the size of the arteriole injected.

This series of events is so well recognized that everyone tries to treat the area of blanch. Some inject it with normal saline, others with a local anesthetic. Some simply rub the area while others have tried rubbing nitroglycerin salve into it. Whether any of these attempts are successful remains to be proven.

Extravasation or injection of an excessively concentrated agent should not cause necrosis of deeper tissues.

Some of the worst ulcers and subsequent pigmentation I have created were in areas where the telangiectasias were quite red in color. These may have represented arteriolar telangiectasias. It is obvious that care should be taken when treating this type of lesion. Treating a tiny test area in an inconspicuous site is a sound idea. Starting with a lesser concentration than usual is also good sense.

Care should also be taken when the telangiectasias, even though blue, are small and form a cluster or mat of fine vessels. There may not be enough normal tissue between the vessels to absorb the minor injury induced in the vein.

Success in sclerotherapy always depends on attention to the myriad details of treatment. Certainly the physician should be sure that the needle lies within the lumen of the vein before injecting the sclerosant. Although blood can be aspirated through a #30 needle the volume is so little in small telangiectasias that none may appear in the syringe even with proper placement of the needle. A #27 needle is often used for injecting telangiectasias and aspiration to verify placement is easier. Should fluid extravasate, as evidenced by the formation of a bleb or local dermal swelling, the injection is terminated.

Post-inflammatory, telangiectatic matting (TM)

This phenomenon is observed not only after injection sclerotherapy but after many kinds of skin injury. The term describes the areas where tiny dilated capillaries have matted together to form a purplish blemish in the skin. Sometimes called a "capillary blush", it is typically 1–2 cm in diameter and develops in areas where telangiectasias have received multiple injections. Matting can also be seen around scars from knee surgery or in areas where microincisional phlebectomy has been performed.

TM is more common on the thigh and occurs in perhaps 10–20% of patients treated for telangiectasias. They have been reported after the use of all the common sclerosants. A number of theories are propounded to explain their development. None are proven. Regardless of cause it is very disturbing for treated patients subsequently to develop a rash of new spider veins.

My feeling is that they develop, especially on the thigh, around typical clusters of spider veins which may be resistant to treatment, thus requiring multiple treatment sessions. These veins are frustrating to the physician and they may be overtreated, i.e. an excessive quantity and concentration of solution may be given in an attempt to eliminate the resistant veins.

The matting does not become apparent until 2–3 weeks after the treatments are begun. The blush is usually more purple than blue and may be mistaken for a bruise by the patient. When the process becomes apparent it is best to stop treating any residual spider veins in the vicinity and let the entire skin area rest. Most of the matted areas will fade and shrink over a period of 3–6 months. If they are still visible I sometimes try a gentle injection if a small feeder vein can be identified. Care should be taken not to create more mats and chase the process from mat to mat. Some vascular lasers have been used with some success when the blush persists and are too small for injections.

While following up a group of patients whose spider veins were treated 15–20 years ago with a 1% STS solution, I noticed that not one of them had any matting or blushing. My only explanation is that only one or two treatments were required in this group and that the matting perhaps is related to the repeated inflammatory response from repeated treatments. The pink blush of TM is shown in Plate 9.

In conclusion, one should treat varicose veins with the strongest solution that does not cause undesired side-effects in order to decrease the number of treatments. This is contrary to the often-repeated idea that one should use the least concentration that is effective in order to avoid side-effects. This is an area which needs further investigation.

Clinical applications

Sodium tetradecyl sulfate

Because of its widespread use STS will be described here in some detail. Since its introduction in 1947 it has proved to be a reliable, predictable, safe and effective sclerosant. It is produced synthetically as a salt of a long-chain fatty acid. As a detergent it has a soapy feel to the fingers. Because it disperses quickly into the blood and can cause hemolysis the vein should be as empty of blood as possible when injections are made. This will also insure that it is not unduly diluted by the blood.

STS has the advantage that its effect is relative to its concentration and remains reproducible at different strengths. Therefore it can be used for almost all sizes of veins. It is supplied in concentrations of 0.2, 0.5, 1 and 3% and can be diluted by the user to his preferred strength. Dilution is with either isotonic saline or sterile water. When multidose vials are used they are usually refrigerated after use although this has been shown to be unnecessary. [5] It is recommended that they be kept away from light. The diluted solutions will remain stable and sterile for at least a month after mixing. Although immediate use is recommended I have used STS from a multidose bottle 2 years after dilution.

As with most sclerosants the strength of the solution should be matched with the type and caliber of vein to be treated. In general the thinner the vein wall (regardless of diameter) the lesser the strength needed to sclerose it. For example a thinned-out 1.5 cm truncal varicosity may only require a 0.5% injection whereas a muscular 4 mm arch vein might need 0.75% to sclerose it.

Although every phlebologist has his own favorite concentration and method of use, certain guidelines can be observed by the less-experienced sclerotherapist.

Common concentrations

- telangiectasias (spider veins)
  0.3–1.0 mm diameter   0.1–0.3%

- varicose reticular v.v. (blue feeder veins)
  1.0–5.0 mm diameter   0.2–0.5%

- non-saphenous varices (e.g. lateral thigh veins)
  0.5–1.0 cm diameter   0.3–0.75%

- saphenous side branches
  0.3–1.0 cm diameter   0.3–0.75%
  1.0–1.5 cm diameter   0.75–1.5%
  >1.5 cm diameter   1.0–3.0%
- saphenous trunks   1.0–3.0%

Polidocanol

POL has the advantage, like STS, of providing a reproducible effect at varying concentrations. At a given percentage POL is about one-half the strength of STS. Thus treating reticular veins with a 0.6% POL is similar to 0.25–0.3% STS.

The tissue effect is almost the same between the two sclerosants. The relative concentrations and dosages for the various veins can be translated from those given for STS. An added advantage of POL is that it was developed as a local anesthetic and seems less painful to many people.

Hypertonic saline

HS was described in the 1920s for treating varicose veins. Its effectiveness in the treatment of telangiectasias was again reported in the mid 1970s, when its use became popular especially with dermatologists. For a while HS with added heparin was commercially available. It was hoped that it would decrease blood trapping. Some physicians still add lidocaine to decrease pain. Evaluations show little advantage to these combinations.

HS is commercially available in concentrations of 23.4 and 12.6%. The greater concentration is effective in closing small varicose reticular veins in the range of 1–2 mm diameter. It is not effective for veins much larger than this or for larger truncal varicosities.

Many phlebologists use the stronger concentrations for treating telangiectasias as well. A useful approach when one is beginning is to inject the reticular veins with stronger and the spider veins with a weaker solution. The 23.4% can be easily diluted and eliminates the need for supplying more than one strength.

HS has some unique and rather unpleasant side-effects. The injection itself can be painful, usually more painful than with the other sclerosants. It can also stimulate a painful cramp in the muscle group beneath the injection site. The reason for these reactions is unknown. Fortunately these side-effects are momentary and a vigorous massage can help relieve the cramp.

Clinical approaches

Several general approaches to injection sclerotherapy have dominated the medical treatment of varicose veins.

The French school of phlebology under the leadership of Tournay established the concept of centrifugal treatment. That is, the treatment is started at the most proximal point of reflux and continued distally. This was performed in a segmental manner from the top of the leg to the bottom. During the development of the method only the varicose veins were injected. Non-invasive testing, especially the use of the Doppler, alerted practitioners to the importance of saphenous reflux. Like other contemporary treatment programs saphenous reflux is eliminated before the varices are treated. Many of the French school obliterate the incompetent saphenous junctions with injections.

Sigg in Switzerland espoused the technique of total sclerosis, in which the entire system of varicosities is injected at one treatment session. Little regard was initially given to the status of the saphenous junctions but as with the French these too are evaluated and treated when necessary. His method emphasized the need to have an empty vein for injection. To obtain this goal a number of needles were introduced into the bulging veins while the patient was standing. Then the leg was elevated and residual blood was drained out through the various needles before injecting the sclerosant.

W.G. Fegan, professor of surgery at Trinity College Dublin, also treated the entire leg during a single session. His method was centripetal wherein the injections were started distally and proceeded proximally with a wrapping applied as the veins were injected. [6]

Prior to the availability of ultrasound examination the saphenous junctions were largely ignored. His concept was that treatment of perforator incompetence would correct or improve saphenous incompetence. Today most physicians practising the Fegan technique close an incompetent SFJ before treating the varicosities.

A major contribution of Fegan's work was to demonstrate the effectiveness of prolonged compression. All varicose veins were treated with injections at the original treatment session. A three layer bandage was then applied whereupon the patient returned to the clinic a week later. Untreated varices were then reinjected. The leg was rewrapped and the wraps left in place for another 5 weeks.

Whether there is a distinct American school of phlebology or not, there is an eclectic approach to the treatment of varicose veins. American surgeons have pioneered the treatment of the more complicated venous problems, pulmonary embolism, venous reconstruction and upper limb deformities. And as American surgeons developed comprehensive stripping methods others were attempting to improve the results of treatment with sclerotherapy. Biegeleisen continued the treatment of spider veins which he started in the 1930s as Orbach advanced the sclerotherapy of large veins using the air block technique. [7,8]

At the same time this author was modifying the Fegan technique to improve the results of stripping and to investigate the use of STS for the treatment of spider veins. [9] Concurrently Foley, a dermatologist, introduced the use of hypertonic saline for the treatment of telangiectasias. [10]

Contemporary sclerotherapy in the USA now recognizes the contribution of each of these schools of phlebology. Workshops, international symposia, improved standards of clinical research and widespread publication of data have improved the quality of sclerotherapy results.

Clinical techniques

Saphenofemoral incompetence

There is now universal agreement that incompetent saphenous trunks should be treated before any attempt is made to treat associated varices. The surgical methods are discussed in Chap. 7. There are many phlebologists in the USA and Europe who obliterate the saphenous veins with sclerotherapy. Unfortunately results reported from different centers vary considerably. Hopefully cooperative efforts among the medical phlebologists will identify which patients can have chemical ablation of the saphenous veins and which require surgical intervention. At this juncture surgery provides the greatest assurance of success.

Telangiectasias (spider veins)

A #30 gauge needle is 0.3 mm in diameter. A vein of this size is simple to cannulate and can easily tolerate a careful injection of 0.3% STS. The fluid will usually flow into the smaller ramifications of the branching venule. Little pressure is required since the fluid is a detergent and races along the vein. Many prefer to use a lesser concentration, although a 0.1% solution is almost isotonic and has little effect when injected. A 0.2% solution may be used but will need more treatments than with 0.3%.

Some phlebologists use a 0.5% concentration in the spider vein. If this is used, only a small volume, barely enough to visibly fill the vein, under minimal pressure, should be used.

My advice to the beginner is to stick to a 0.3% or lesser concentration and find out how it works before moving to a higher dosage. The results of treating the blue vein-spider vein complex are shown in Plate 10.

When telangiectasias stretch above 1 mm in diameter they become very thin-walled. This type of telangiectasia is seen on the leg when the process has been present for many years. They are also seen on the ankle and foot and represent the corona phlebectatica ("blue blebs" in our dictionary). Because of their thin walls they will ulcerate if too-strong a solution is used. A 0.25–0.3% STS solution is usually strong enough to sclerose them but mild enough not to ulcerate them. [11]

These larger spider veins are prone to trap blood after injection with resultant pigmentation. They should be compressed if at all possible to decrease thrombosis.

Reticular (blue) veins

These dermal veins measure 1–5 mm in diameter. My preference is to inject all of them with a 0.3–0.5% STS or 0.75% POL solution. These larger veins may respond to a lesser concentration but will require more treatments. One wants to keep the number of treatments to a minimum.

Reticular veins are quite different from the spider vein both in structure and in response to treatment. They are thicker-walled with more muscular fibers and lie in a deeper cuticular or subcuticular position. They can therefore tolerate a stronger injection without the adverse side-effects seen in the spider veins. In spite of their thicker construction they respond quickly to sclerotherapy and may require fewer treatments to effect closure than their secondary spider veins.

Non-saphenous varicosities

The lateral thigh and calf veins are examples of veins responsive to sclerotherapy. When incompetent they are usually associated with other varicose reticular veins. They appear to be independent of the saphenous veins but may be connected with varicose saphenous tributaries and measure 0.5–0.8 mm in diameter. They are often attached to the anterior or lateral accessory saphenous vein or the posterior thigh vein.

The larger veins are frequently part of the complex of incompetent reticular veins which feed the telangiectasias of the thigh and calf. They are under minimal venous hypertension and are relatively thin-walled, making them "sclerosensitive".

A solution of 0.3–0.5% STS is again used for these veins. They may respond to treatment more quickly than their associated spider veins, possibly in two or three sessions.

Truncal varicosities/saphenous tributaries

We have mentioned before that the concentration for use depends primarily on the size and wall thickness of the vein treated. Most of the saphenous tributaries in their normal state are less than 1 cm in diameter. As they stretch under pressure the wall thins out. This makes them more "sclerosensitive".

Most truncal varicosities will respond well to solutions of 0.5–1.5%. A concentration less than 1.0% will suffice in most cases. Higher doses are more likely to cause a perivenitis and pigmentation. When the vein is deeper these changes may not be quite so apparent. Such a treatment program can be observed in Plate 11.

For thicker veins such as arch veins or segments of the saphenous veins, a concentration of 1.0–3.0% may be required for closure. Some of the varices on the foot and ankle can be quite thick-walled and require a concentration of 1% or more.

My tendency through the years has been to decrease the concentrations of sclerosants used. In my early experience 3% STS was used for all larger veins and 1% for smaller veins including spider veins. The number of ulcers and prolonged pigmentation was measurably greater with that regimen.

On the other hand a dose strong enough to shed the endothelium and disturb the vein wall should be used the first time around. If repeated lighter doses are used the vein may become resistant to treatment, thrombosing and recanalizing with each treatment attempt rather than sclerosing.

However, the beginner should perform the safest

treatment. That is to say he should use the smallest effective concentration and find out its effect before trying higher concentrations which may allow fewer treatment sessions.

When treating smaller veins the use of a mild sclerosant may be frustrating to patient and doctor because little effect is noted at first. They think it is not working and stop treatments. The vein simply needs more treatments.

Spider veins on the face and other bodily parts can be treated with sclerotherapy. Even those secondary to radiotherapy are responsive. The newer vascular lasers may possibly do a better job.

Methods/materials

Reusable glass syringes are popular with Europeans and some Americans because the plunger moves easily to aspirate blood to verify placement. With the relatively low cost of disposables and the litigious environment in which we work disposables are recommended. Besides, nursing staff hate to clean and sterilize glass syringes.

For most injections a 3 ml plastic syringe fits the hand nicely. I use a #20–23 gauge needle to draw up the solution. For blue veins and spider veins I use a #30 for the injections. I seldom aspirate to confirm an intravascular position although this can be done through the #30. The spider is so close to the skin surface that visual confirmation of position is possible.

The barrel is held with the index and third fingers, like a cigarette. The thumb depresses the plunger. With the bevel up the needle is bent at the hub approximately 20 degrees. This permits the length of the needle to lie on the skin as its tip slides into the vein. This position provides the greatest support for the hand and needle.

Other positions for holding the syringe should be practised. Those using glass syringes usually hold the barrel like a pool cue and manipulate the plunger with the little finger. When I started experimenting on spider vein injections I held the barrel between thumb and third finger and depressed the plunger with the index finger. This position can be useful at times to inject a vein in a difficult place. [12] These techniques are seen in Fig. 8.1.

Remember the smaller the syringe the greater is the pressure which can be generated with the same finger pressure. Thus a 1 ml tuberculin syringe can produce an enormous pressure which can burst a tiny vein with little apparent push.

A small injection is made and continued if the vein accepts the fluid. If the needle is not in the vein a small bleb rises in the skin. The injection is stopped.

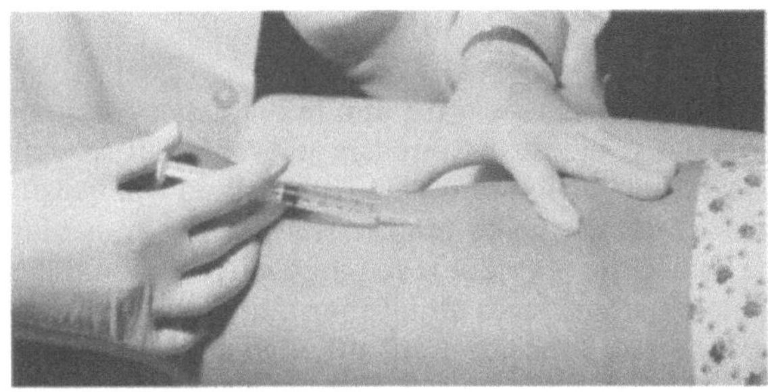

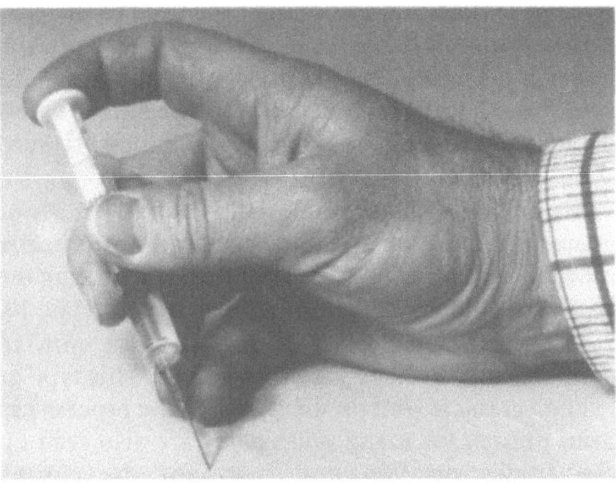

Figure 8.1 Two methods of holding the injecting syringe are shown. The position in the upper photograph is probably the most widely used technique and allows the needle to lie on the skin surface as it is advanced. The other hand stretches the skin, a maneuver necessary regardless of the syringe position. The lower photograph was taken from the original article describing the use of sodium tetradecyl sulfate in the treatment of spider veins [12]. It is a useful alternative for difficult vein positions.

In almost all cases the needle is too deep, having penetrated the back wall of the vein. In this situation the vein will frequently accept fluid if slight pressure is applied as the needle is slowly withdrawn from the vein.

When injecting more concentrated solutions in larger veins I attach a #27 needle which allows easy aspiration for verification of proper needle placement.

Often the needle can be seen to "pop" into a larger vein as it is advanced through the skin. The skin surface is slightly tethered by the movement of the needle through it. This depression is released as the needle pops into the lumen.

Tourniquet

Many physicians place a tourniquet above the site of injection in hopes of distending the vein. This concept is fallacious because varicose veins are distended by reflux from above the injection site, not from below. The tourniquet may actually block the filling of the varix.

One effective method for filling the varices is to place a tourniquet around the thigh and inflate it to 70 mmHg to occlude the deep and superficial veins. This is done in the sitting or prone position. The varices quickly distend, the needle is inserted, the tourniquet released and the injection made.

Position

It has been a tradition to perform injections with the patient standing to distend the veins. There are two problems with this technique. First, many patients faint. Secondly, the sclerosant is unnecessarily diluted in this position. It is essential to have the vein as empty of blood as possible.

There are other better methods of distending the veins and positioning the needle correctly. A popular technique has the patient standing. Then a butterfly needle(s) is inserted with the needle taped tangentially to the skin. A regular needle and syringe can be attached in the same way. The patient lies down, the leg is elevated to empty it of blood and the injection made through the butterfly needle.

To maintain a completely empty vessel a tourniquet is placed distal to the needle so that no more blood flows into the proximal vein.

Fegan made a habit of isolating the segment of vein with his fingers. Once the needle is in place, the leg is elevated and a finger placed on either side of the needle and residual blood milked away from it. The fingers are left in place for a few moments after injection to permit contact of solution with the vein endothelium. Shadeck has recently observed with the duplex scanner that the solution may float on a layer of blood. He taps the vein intermittently with his finger to better distribute the solution (personal communication).

Urtication

For superficial injections the skin reacts to the injection in a rather uniform manner. The immediate appearance is that of an insect bite or a positive allergy skin test. There is a raised whitish *wheal* with a surrounding *flare* in the skin. The wheal is a localized hive probably from histamine release. Sometimes when a large volume of fluid is injected in a larger reticular vein the entire injection tract will urticate. Deeper veins show little surface reaction to the injection and are less painful. Urtication can develop with the use of any of the sclerosants, even hypertonic saline. Should hives become a problem or if there are other histamine-release problems such as headache, these

can be controlled by the use of oral antihistamines taken before the treatment.

Pain

The sensory response to injections is varied. The response seems to vary according to the perceptions of the patient and his particular "pain threshold".

Some report excruciating pain, especially from hypertonic saline. This may be accompanied with muscle cramps. Little cramping is reported using other sclerosants.

The needle insertion is quite painless even for the "needleophobic". Often a #30 needle is not felt at all. However, most patients complain of burning and stinging when the fluid is injected. If a little fluid extravasates during an otherwise successful injection the patient may feel added discomfort. The injection is stopped.

Pain, burning or stinging are more pronounced the more superficial the veins are in the skin. Thus injecting spider telangiectasias is more painful than injecting a larger subcutaneous varicosity. There is a concentration of tiny nerve endings in the upper dermis where the spider veins reside.

Rubbing the injected area will usually help diminish the painful response. Severe pain should subside after 10–15 s and disappear within 4–5 min.

As I have stated before I first tried treating spider veins in the early 1970s (without the benefit of a tutor) by injecting them with a 1% STS solution. The shots were quite painful for each patient but followed the above guidelines. Many tiny ulcerations formed. Many of these patients 10–15 years later still have an area of slight depigmentation at the ulcer site, although it is distinctly different from the scars observed with more recent treatment methods. A few, especially around the ankles, still have a vague halo of pigment at the ulcer site.

It is also of interest that there are never any new spider veins in the exact area originally treated. It is as if the skin were sterilized of neogenesis. New spider veins develop only in adjacent areas.

Compression

The are many phlebologists who use no compression after injecting varicose veins. On the other hand there are many phlebologists who believe that every injected vein should be compressed. This latter view may well be true although I personally tend to use less compression than many other phlebologists.

Although compression has been used sporadically for 70 years there was little scientific basis for its use. Everyone agrees that compression helps to decrease post-injection pain and thrombus formation but it was Fegan who first demonstrated with biopsies the advantages of continued compression. [1] The histologic examinations showed that continued compression for 5 weeks diminished thrombus formation and enhanced fibrocytic migration between the compressed vein walls.

Three major questions have yet to be resolved concerning the use of compression: what type of compression is best, how much compression is necessary, and how long should the compression be maintained to obtain maximum benefit?

Ideally the compression should be strong enough to collapse the vein, to express residual blood and to discourage thrombosis. A more complete discussion of compression methods is presented in Chap. 9.

Truncal varicose veins

It is essential to use compression with these larger varicose veins. In the past when they were treated solely by sclerotherapy below knee hosiery, either 20–30 mmHg or 30–40 mmHg were used. Thigh high stockings were also used when thigh veins were treated.

When microincisional phlebectomy was initiated we compared the results of thigh vein sclerotherapy to phlebectomy. For larger thigh varicosities phlebectomy gave superior results because of the difficulty of compressing the thigh. Our current approach is to phlebectomize the larger truncal varicosities, especially those on the thigh, and inject the smaller residuals.

Compression is used for both treatment modalities. Depending on the size and shape of the thighs, wrapping or compression bandaging is used for 3 days post-operatively. The calf may be wrapped or stockings applied. Compression for a week has given very satisfactory results.

Reticular veins

In general I do not compress the common variety of varicose reticular veins 1–2 mm in diameter. They seldom cause blood trapping or pigmentation. However, when they have been present for many years and are dilated more than 5 mm they should be compressed for at least a week. In this state they are thin-walled and tend to trap blood and become pigmented like truncal varicosities of the same size.

Telangiectasias

Only one study has tested the effect of compression hosiery on injected telangiectasias. The major finding suggested a decrease in pigmentation and local swelling.

I do not routinely compress this group although members of our clinic find that there is less pain and perhaps less blood trapping when the legs are compressed. Certainly a patient who has exaggerated urtication and pain will appreciate overnight compression. Schultz-Ehrenburg claims that a lower grade of elastic hosiery, e.g. 20–30 mmHg, can provide as effective a control of cutaneous venous hypertension as higher graded stockings (personal communication).

Comments

Injection sclerotherapy holds a rightful place in the treatment of varicose and telangiectatic veins. Our collective experience and controlled studies have given us more scientific information and fewer anecdotal comments on which to base our treatments.

The addition of compression has improved our results when compared to those reported in earlier decades. At the same time the availability of new sclerosing agents allows us to individualize the treatments to match the vein problem of the patient. Although an occasional mild complication or side-effect seems to be inevitable, most can now be avoided. Careful attention to the use of appropriate sclerosants and to the details of technique should avoid most complications and insure successful treatment results.

The report of a recent international consensus conference on sclerotherapy should be required reading for anyone interested in learning this technique. [13]

Manufacturing sources of sclerosants

Sodium tetradecyl sulfate

- Sotradecol, Wyeth-Ayerst Laboratories, Philadelphia, PA, USA
- Fibro-Vein, STD Pharmaceutical Products Ltd, Hereford, UK
- Thromboject, Omega Laboratories Ltd, Montreal, Canada

Polidocanol

- Aethoxysklerol, Chemische Fabrik Kreussler AG, Wiesbaden, Germany
- Sclerovein, Resinag AG, Schwyz, Switzerland
- Aetoxisclerol, Laboratoires Pharmaceutiques Dexo, SA, Nanterre, France

Sodium morrhuate

- Scleromate, Palisades Pharmaceutical Inc., Tenafly, NJ, USA
- generic, American Regent Laboratories, Shirley, NY, USA

Ethanolamine oleate

- Ethamolin, Reed & Carnick, Jersey City, NJ, USA
- generic, Block Drug Co., Piscataway, NJ, USA

Hypertonic saline

- many manufacturers

Hypertonic saline/hypertonic dextrose

- Sclerodex, Omega Laboratories Ltd, Montreal, Canada

Chromated glycerin

- Scleremo, Laboratories E. Bouteille, Lomoges, France

- Chromex, Omega Laboratories Ltd, Montreal, Canada

References

1. Fegan WG (1963) Continuous compression technique of injecting varicose veins. Lancet 2:109–113
2. Goldman MP (1995) Sclerotherapy, Treatment of Varicose and Telangiectatic Leg Veins, 2nd edn. Mosby, St Louis
3. Tretbar LL, Pattisson PH (1970) Injection–compression treatment of varicose veins. Am J Surg 120:539–541
4. Tretbar LL (1989) Injection sclerotherapy for spider telangiectasias: a 20-year experience with sodium tetradecyl sulfate. J Dermatol Surg Oncol 15:223–225
5. Sadick NS, Farber B (1993) A microbiologic study of diluted sclerotherapy solutions. J Dermatol Surg Oncol 19:450–454
6. Fegan WG (1967) Varicose veins, compression sclerotherapy. Charles C Thomas, Springfield
7. Biegeleisen HI (1933) The evaluation of sodium morrhuate therapy in varicose veins: a critical study. Surg Gynecol Obstet 57:696–699
8. Orbach EJ (1944) Sclerotherapy of varicose veins: utilization of intravenous air block. Am J Surg 66:362–667
9. Pattisson PH, Tretbar LL (1971) The injection treatment of varicose veins: a follow-up study of 264 patients. Vasc Surg 5:1–5
10. Foley WT (1975) The eradication of venous blemishes. Cutis 15:665–668
11. Tretbar LL (1996) Treatment of small bleeding varicose veins with injection sclerotherapy. Dermatol Surg 22:78–80
12. Tretbar LL (1978) Spider angiomata: treatment with sclerosant injections. J Kans Med Soc 79:198–201
13. Baccaglini U, Spreafico G, Castoro C, Sorrentino P eds (1997) Consensus conference on sclerotherapy of varicose veins of the lower limbs. Phlebology 12:2–16

CHAPTER 9

Complications of Chronic Venous Insufficiency

The major complications of chronic, uncompensated venous insufficiency encompass a distinctive series of dermatologic changes usually developing in the skin and subcutaneous tissues of the lower leg and ankle. These changes develop slowly over a period of years and include ulceration, liposclerosis, edema, pigmentation, eczematoid dermatitis and white atrophy. Symptoms of intense itching, stinging, burning, aching, throbbing and actual pain may accompany the anatomic changes.

Traditionally the changes, particularly ulcerations, were thought to be late sequelae of DVT. The terms commonly used to describe these conditions were the "post-phlebitic leg" or "post-thrombotic syndrome". We now know that all of the chronic changes and complications found in the so-called post-thrombotic syndrome can develop as a result of pure superficial venous insufficiency.

It is also clear that the treatment of secondary varicose veins can improve the functional aspects of deep venous insufficiency by eliminating the continued overload of refluxing blood.

Cutaneous complications

Gaiter area

For some unknown reason the area of the lower calf and ankle, known as the "gaiter area", is the region where most of the chronic cutaneous changes occur. A gaiter is a piece of clothing covering the lower trousers, much like spats, and worn over the ankle and shoe by the military, bishops and Boy Scout color

guards. Gaiters are now popular with skiers to keep snow out of their boots.

Usually the foot is not affected by CVH even though the hydrostatic pressure is greater here. One can speculate that the local ambulatory pressure may be minimized by the foot pump. The foot pump is dead-ended so that the blood has no place to go but upward and is continuously emptied by walking.

A traditional answer for the exaggerated skin changes in the gaiter area is that there are incompetent Cockett's perforating veins lying beneath this area which transmit added pressure to the skin and subcutaneous tissues. Our improved testing methods especially color ultrasonography may help to answer this question. The *gaiter area* demonstrates the changes of CVI in Fig. 9.1.

Lipodermatosclerosis

This term, coined by Bernand [1], describes the progressive fibrotic changes of the skin and subcutaneous fat induced by chronic venous hypertension. These changes were also described by Trendelenburg in 1891. The changes are usually confined to the gaiter area where the skin becomes indurated, firm and shiny. The subcutaneous fat becomes thickened and hard, a condition similar to that seen with post-traumatic fat necrosis. Although the tissues are originally thickened they gradually contract and the diameter of the ankle narrows.

Varicose veins within this fibrotic skin appear as canyons. For some unknown reason the skin above the vein may not be pigmented even though the surrounding skin is dark.

Lipodermatosclerosis can have an acute phase

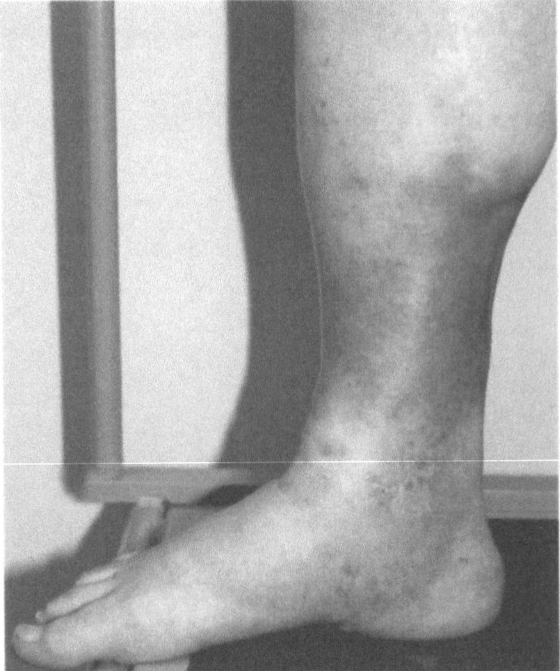

Figure 9.1 Many of the characteristic changes of chronic venous insufficiency are seen here. The skin of the gaiter area has been thickened, pigmented and narrowed. The foot has been spared these changes. In this case there was gross incompetence of the greater saphenous vein. Stripping and phlebectomy and continued compression have improved these changes over a 3 year period.

wherein a relatively normal area of skin is affected. The patient complains of a painful, hot, burning area on the calf or ankle which is usually tender to the touch. Clear fluid, probably lymph, may weep from the turgid skin. It is bright red or brownish in color and may be mistaken as a case of acute cellulitis. Unless there is a superimposed infection antibiotics fail to improve the condition.

It is important to distinguish between an episode of acute liposclerosis and acute thrombophlebitis. Phlebitis is more localized with a distinctive tender cord beneath. Anticoagulation has no place in the treatment of liposclerosis. Acute liposclerosis usually improves with compression and anti-inflammatory medication but may progress into the chronic form.

Pigmentation

Early in the liposclerotic process the skin of the gaiter area is covered with reddish petechiae. Gradually the skin darkens, often with hemosiderin deposits forming a brown pigment. Although most of the discoloration is a result of blood breakdown, some may be due to melanin stimulation as well.

An interesting variation to this finding is represented in Fig. 9.2.

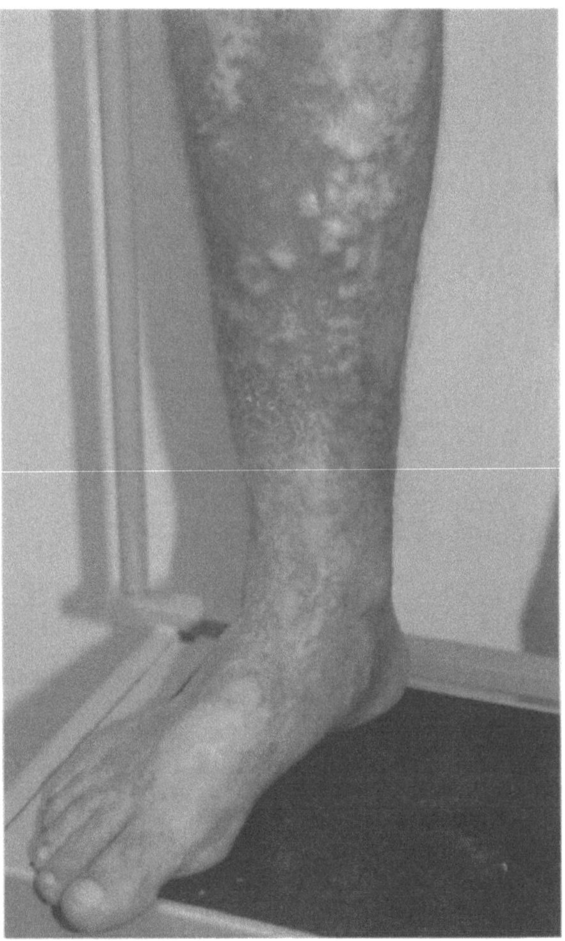

Figure 9.2 In this patient the gaiter area shows the typical changes of chronic venous insufficiency: thickening, narrowing and pigmentation. There is also a dry scaly dermatitis on the surface. However, the skin directly over the large varicose veins is *depigmented*. No one has yet explained this curious phenomenon.

White atrophy

White atrophy, *atrophie blanche* in French, is another typical skin change found with CVI. The term perfectly describes the appearance of the skin. It is both white and atrophic. Well-circumscribed areas of epithelium are depigmented and pale because there are no capillaries to impart a normal pink color to the surface. This phenomenon has been presented in Plate 1.

White atrophy usually represents the scars of healed venous ulcers. The skin lesions are areas which have been damaged and heal in an ischemic environment. There may also be areas of pale atrophic skin which have not been ulcerated. This skin has had ischemic damage while the integrity of the epithelium has been maintained. In the absence of nutritive capillaries the skin remains ischemic; the tissue is fragile and susceptible to minor trauma.

Eczema

An eczematous dermatitis often develops during the process. In the chronic state the skin surface tends to be dry and flaky but may become inflamed with an acute episode of liposclerosis.

Not only do eczematoid changes develop spontaneously but a secondary neurodermatitis is frequently observed. This is a result of the vigorous scratching which accompanies the intense itching. The skin may actually be excoriated by the fingernails as well. This particular dermatologic change can be differentiated from other primary causes by the fact that the dermatitis often follows the course of the pruritic vein.

Edema

Swelling is a common feature of CVI, especially when there is chronic deep venous insufficiency. Edema may be one of the first signs of advancing venous insufficiency. Early the edema may only be seen from behind where there is fluid on either side of the Achilles tendon. As the swelling continues it encompasses the ankle but may not involve the foot itself. During the initial stages of insufficiency the edema fluid is simply an increased amount of interstitial fluid which has seeped from the venules. The fluid is relatively low in protein content and usually disappears overnight with elevation; however, as the process develops elevation may not completely relieve the swelling. Although prolonged venous insufficiency can develop lymphedema there is little mistaking true primary or secondary lymphedema. Plate 12 illustrates a well-advanced case of CVI due to superficial disease. This condition is contrasted in Plate 13 which demonstrates pure lymphedema of a hereditary nature.

Venous ulceration

Ulceration is the final insult to the skin. The ulcers are properly called "chronic venous ulcers" and are found in the gaiter area usually originating on the medial ankle just above the malleolus, although they may be seen in any area of the lower leg. They may become circumferential or develop in atypical areas. The differential diagnosis is seldom difficult because there are other stigmata of chronic venous disease, pigmentation, liposclerosis, thickening and narrowing of the skin. A typical, deep, sharply demarcated venous ulcer is seen in Fig. 9.3.

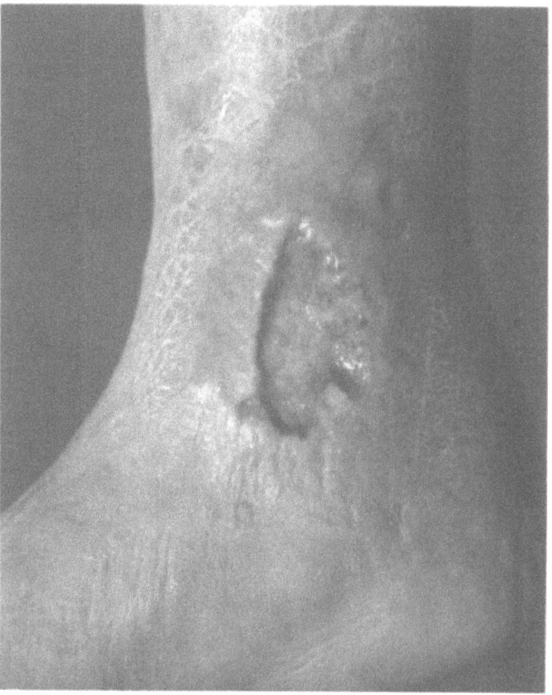

Figure 9.3 This patient was one of the unfortunate patients during the 1960s who had vena caval interruption to prevent pulmonary embolization from a DVT. He was plagued with recurring ulcerations for more than 20 years. Continued compression therapy halted the ulcerative process and improved his venous claudication.

Pathogenesis of venous ulceration

The process by which chronic venous disease causes ulcers provides an unending source of research, speculation, investigation and discussion. As yet there is no clear evidence of causation although there are many findings of altered physiologic, hematologic, histologic and immunologic function.

Early in this century Homans introduced the term "venous stasis ulcer". [2] The concept has colored our thinking for many generations and led to the idea that stagnant blood in the varicose veins near the skin resulted in tissue anoxia and death. He further observed the association of incompetent perforating veins from previous DVT and emphasized their importance in the development of the "post-phlebitic leg". Investigators have since demonstrated not only an accelerated blood flow but a higher oxygen tension in the venous blood of legs with ulcers than in normal legs. [3,4] These findings were thought by some to support the stasis theory by suggesting that oxygen was not transmitted to the skin and remained in the venous blood.

Later speculators suggested that the increased flow and elevated oxygen levels in the venous blood of patients with CVI could be explained by "pathological shunting" through arteriovenous fistulae. Again the skin was thought to be deprived of oxygen and anoxic tissue death ensued. These pathologic arteriovenous fistulae have yet to be demonstrated although they have been assiduously sought for.

Then there was the idea that chronic edema deprived the tissues of proper oxygen exchange. This idea too has not been proven. However, Browse and Bernand [5], on histologic examination of tissues around venous ulcers, discovered a pericapillary cuff of fibrin. They suggested that the "fibrin cuffs", demonstrated both histochemically and immunochemically, might have developed from increased capillary leakage of plasma proteins which included plasminogen. These cuffs certainly exist, perhaps as a result of reduced fibrinolytic activity which has been found in the entire limbs of these patients. That these fibrin cuffs can restrict oxygen exchange in the tissues has not been proven.

Another concept to explain ulceration indicts the WBC as the villain. There are numerous studies which show trapping of WBCs in the lower limb in patients with CVI. Schmid-Schonbein [6] has demonstrated how WBCs adhere to the venular wall and because of their relatively larger size block the flow of RBCs. It would be too simplistic to suggest that this would impair oxygen exchange in the skin.

However, it is well recognized that increased WBC adherence to endothelium is a characteristic of acute inflammation. Coleridge Smith and associates [7] advance a hypothesis to explain the cellular damage of liposclerosis and ulceration. They propose that "reduced capillary flow rates lead to increased WBC adhesion to the endothelium." This has two consequences. An effective reduction in capillary caliber leads to further reduced flow and eventual occlusion of the vessel. Adherence also results in activation of both the WBC and the endothelial cell; the latter releases chemotactic factors attracting further WBCs, while the activated neutrophils themselves degranulate and discharge proteolytic enzymes and a variety of free radicals which damage the endothelial membrane. The capillary as a result becomes "leaky", and a protein- and fibrin-rich exudate escapes into the extravascular space" [8]. These substances have non-specific destructive effects on lipid membranes, proteins and many connective tissue compounds.

He further reminds us of the process called the "Schwarzmann reaction" in which an inflammatory infiltrate sensitizes the local tissue. Minor trauma or infection then activates the sensitized cells and a rapidly necrotizing destruction of the skin ensues.

Venous ulcers seem to develop in such a fashion. The atrophic liposclerotic area may be the time bomb waiting for a detonator. Minor trauma often triggers the explosion within the tissues and an ulcer suddenly appears. Although this theory is attractive and more than plausible it remains to be proven as do the other theories of causation.

Superficial versus deep insufficiency

When venous failure is purely superficial there may be few long-term effects except perhaps for the development of varicose veins. In this situation the muscle pumps can empty the excessive blood volume. Ambulatory venous pressure remains normal and the progressive changes of venous hypertension are avoided.

However, there are many instances where legs demonstrating all of the changes of CVI, dermato-sclerosis, pigmentation and ulceration, show no evidence of DVT or deep venous insufficiency. Estimates of these changes from superficial disease range from 25 to 65%. We must assume that in these cases the calf pump cannot keep up with the increasing venous overload of superficial reflux. Venous hypertension ensues and progressive skin changes develop in the lower leg. Many of these ulcers appear at the end of the long saphenous vein as if it were a garden hose transmitting the pressure to the ankle.

There are some differences in the cutaneous complications arising from superficial insufficiency and in those from deep insufficiency. Those with superficial disease usually have less swelling than those with deep insufficiency. Ulcerations are more shallow and smaller in diameter. Pigmentation may be more localized over the surface veins and liposclerosis may be less advanced.

There are some phlebologists who do not believe that these changes of CVI can develop with purely superficial venous incompetence. They maintain that there must be at least some other incompetence such as incompetent perforating veins in the gaiter area. This controversy too remains to be settled.

The significance of CVI with a normal deep venous system is that the causes of superficial CVI, incompetent saphenous trunk or incompetent perforating veins can be corrected. Contrary to the problems of deep venous insufficiency, which have little chance of being corrected, the progressive nature of the superficial disease can be halted. It is therefore obligatory for the phlebologist to identify this group of patients. In the past most patients with skin problems or ulcerations were assumed to have deep venous insufficiency, even without testing, and relegated to a life-time of compression hose, as illustrated by the patient shown in Fig. 3.2 and Plate 12.

Evaluation

We perform as complete a vascular evaluation as seems appropriate to determine the status of the deep and superficial systems. The patient is examined in the standing position and often requires support such as a walker.

If there is massive swelling of the lower leg with all of the associated skin changes one strongly suspects this to be a true post-phlebitic leg, i.e. post-DVT. Doppler examination of the popliteal vein usually reveals free reflux with augmentation and sometimes a positive Valsalva. Often the LSV is incompetent as well. A duplex scan is obligatory for a proper evaluation of the deep system.

Evaluation of the arterial system is equally important because ischemic arterial ulcers can coexist with venous disease. One must be cautious too that compression needed for treatment does not compromise arterial flow. Arterial insufficiency may be excluded by clinical examination and by the brachial/ankle arterial pressure ratio. This is a comparison of arterial blood pressures obtained in the arm to the pressure measured in the ankle. The technique of this test is described in Chap. 4.

A ratio greater than 0.8 is generally considered normal. When the leg is swollen an arterial pressure may not be easily obtained using the usual cuff. A larger cuff slowly inflated can compress the artery. The Doppler is essential for hearing blood flow in the posterior tibial artery. From a practical aspect, if the posterior tibial artery pulse can be felt with the fingers and heard with the Doppler the arterial circulation is probably adequate.

A careful Doppler examination of the ulcer and surrounding tissue is also enlightening. The ulcer is usually quite painful and sensitive to touch; however, a large glob of gel can be placed in the ulcer bed and the probes held just above the tissue surface. In most cases reflux is heard beneath the ulcer. We were taught that there was always an incompetent perforating vein beneath the ulcer. This may or may not be true. In many instances flow is heard beneath the ulcer and may be from a varicose vein. Doppler examination of an atypical lateral ulcer is shown in Fig. 9.4.

Treatment of the ulcer is initiated at the first visit even though testing may not be complete or surgical treatment is planned.

Treatment of chronic venous ulcers

Although there is not always agreement about many of the details of treatment, most phlebologists agree

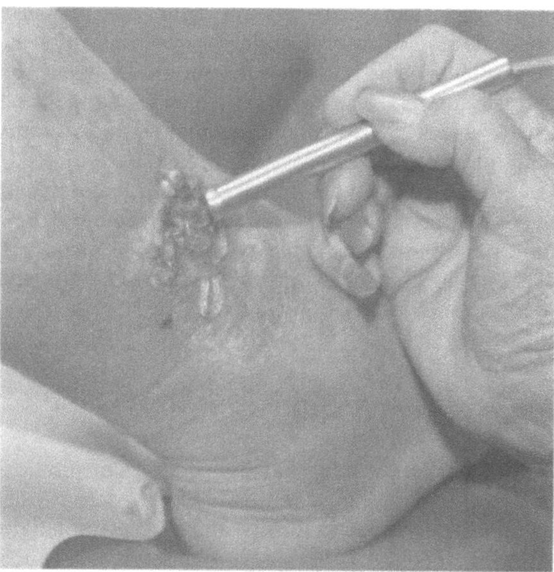

Figure 9.4 Doppler interrogation of this ulcer showed that there was a direct venous link between it and a totally incompetent lesser saphenous vein. The results of compressive treatment are seen in Plate 15.

with the principles of treatment. Some objectives of treatment are:

- reduction of venous hypertension
- reduction and control of edema
- local treatment of ulcers
- treatment of infection
- care of peri-ulcer skin

Reduction of venous hypertension

Many patients appear in our clinic having had only topical treatment of their ulcers, and little or no attention paid to the underlying venous disease.

Venous hypertension is initially controlled with compression. Direct surgical treatment of incompetent saphenous trunks, their associated varicose veins and incompetent perforating veins is then essential. This decreases venous hypertension by decreasing reflux and thereby decreases transmural pressure. My personal belief is that any varicose vein associated with ulcers, whether from deep or superficial insufficiency, should be treated. We have seen remarkable improvement in deep venous function after treatment of secondary varicosities.

Reduction and control of edema

When feasible, bed rest with the legs sharply elevated is the best method of reducing edema. It is almost impossible to reduce edema with compression methods alone. Any type or degree of elevation of the legs allows gravity to withdraw fluid from the extravascular compartment. Much of the fluid found in late stages of CVI is lymphedema which contains a higher protein concentration than venous fluid. If the other aspects of treatment are to be successful it may be necessary to put the patient to bed for a few days before initiating other types of edema control. Treating leg ulcers has always been a problem of the medical profession as shown in Fig. 9.5.

Manual lymph drainage (MLD)

MLD is part of a comprehensive program of physical therapy for controlling edema and lymphedema. MLD itself was developed in Europe and consists of a light stroking massage. It opens lymphatic vessels which have been closed by spasm or those which surround an obstructed area of lymphatic drainage. The light massage is supplemented by wrapping, exercise and compression. It is widely used in Europe and is available in some American lymphedema treatment centers.

Compression

Compression has been used for centuries to treat leg ulcers. Even today it is the mainstay of treatment. Although there has been considerable study of the effects of compression, its mechanism of action still remains unknown.

External compression of course decreases transmural pressure gradients, perhaps forcing some free fluid back into the veins or preventing leakage. Some believe it helps alter the fibrin/fibrinogen ratio which may decrease interstitial fluid and improve oxygen exchange.

There are four approaches to compression:

- wrapping with elastic bandages
- wrapping with limited stretch bandages
- graduated compression hose
- pneumatic pumping

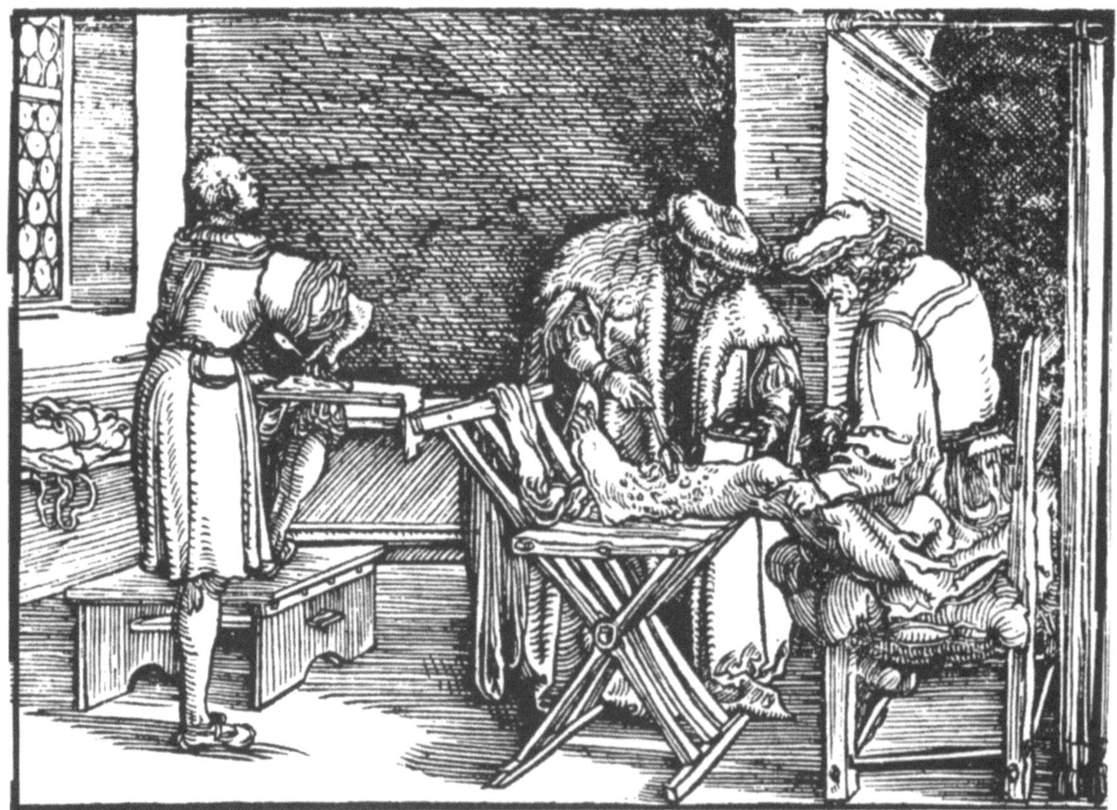

Figure 9.5 This woodcut of 1584, attributed to Holbein, is probably by Hans Weitz. The physician, with his academic cap and gown, must be more than a mere barber-surgeon. His treatment of an ulcer on an edematous leg appears to cause little discomfort to the patient. The apprentice prepares a poltice on his knee board; linen wrappings are draped nearby.

Elastic bandages

Elastic wrappings are widely known to most sports advocates since we use them to wrap sprained ankles and wrists. They are more popular in the USA than in other countries for compressing legs; they are thought to be effective in all positions and for longer periods. They are also popular because they are easy to apply over other bandages and conform to awkward body shapes.

The elastic variety can stretch up to 150% or more of their initial length. A presumed advantage is that as swelling recedes the bandage shrinks with it. However, when a person walks the wrappings stretch with the expansion of the muscles and lose part of their compressive force. If worn at night they must be loosened or removed to avoid their continued compression.

Many physicians prefer to keep the leg wrapped during the healing of the ulcer rather than to use hosiery, since (i) the pressure gradients can be more precisely adjusted and (ii) it is easier to change ulcer dressings when wearing the bandage, especially during the early exudative stages.

Limited stretch bandages

Unlike stretch bandages, limited or short stretch bandages can only be stretched 70–80% of their length. They function somewhat like the muscular fascia. The wrapping envelops the leg with only moderate compression of its own. During exercise the expansion of the muscles presses against the inelastic wrap. An advantage of this system is that they can be worn at night, when there is minimal muscular activity. Excess compression is avoided, which sometimes occurs with elastic wraps.

A slight disadvantage occurs when massive edema is being treated. As the degree of swelling decreases with walking the bandage loosens and must be rewrapped. Some patients do not like to use them because they do not conform to the contours of the leg as well as the purely elastic wraps. Wrapping requires a more precise technique to prevent them from slipping and falling down.

From a technical viewpoint Neumann has presented some very convincing evidence as to the superiority of limited stretch wrappings. [9] He measured the interface pressure, that is the pressure between the skin and bandage, of a short stretch and an elastic bandage in patients at rest and during exercise. The principal findings were that the limited stretch wrappings gave better compression during the exercise phase of the protocol and could be worn at rest. Figure

9.6 shows a patient who is wrapping an edematous arm with layers of inelastic bandage.

Graduated compression hosiery

The term "graduated compression" means that the compression created by the hosiery is not uniform but graduated throughout the length of the stocking. A stocking designated as 20–30 mmHg will provide about 30 mmHg compression at the level of the ankle and 20 mmHg compression at the calf. This graduation encourages the flow of fluid from the greater to the lesser pressure, that is, from lower to higher.

Although good comparative studies have not been done, most clinicians have found that graduated compression hose are essential for proper treatment. For advanced venous insufficiency the patient will usually require hosiery of at least 30–40 mmHg in strength. Some patients will require 40–50 mmHg to reduce or maintain control of edema. One must be careful in advising people to wear the stronger hose. They are difficult at best for most people to put on. Even with the new "valet" frames which assist in pulling on the hose, there are many patients who simply refuse to wear them. In this circumstance lighter hose are better than no hose at all.

To solve this problem many patients prefer the "two-stocking technique" of compression. Here two lighter stockings are worn, one over the other. For example two 20 mmHg hose will provide almost 40 mmHg total pressure. The advantage is that they are easier to pull on, one over the other. Also when swelling recedes only one pair may be necessary.

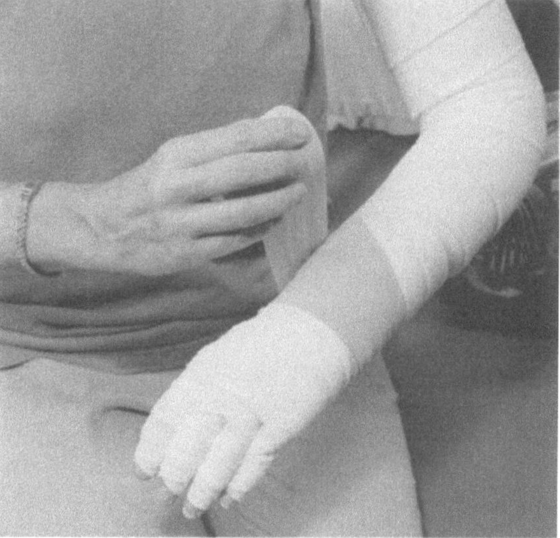

Figure 9.6 The treatment of arm edema is no different from that of leg edema. This patient had edema secondary to axillary irradiation. Her treatment consisted of manual lymph drainage, wrapping and compression garments. Similar treatments are given to those patients with edema of the legs.

For people with deep venous insufficiency compression hose must be worn indefinitely. No one knows with certainty whether the wearing of them decreases the recurrence of ulceration although everyone agrees that it does.

For the person with minimal swelling from superficial disease continued compression may not be necessary after the surface disease has been treated completely. Unfortunately most patients with ulcers already have the other dermatologic changes of CVI and may benefit from continued compression. [10]

Intermittent pneumatic compression

It has been shown in a number of studies that the addition of pneumatic pumping to the standard compression method hastens the healing of ulcers. These devices are comprised of a plastic boot of varying lengths which is attached to a pneumatic pump. A typical treatment approach uses a graduated pneumatic compression device that applies a graduated compression greatest at the foot, which decreases as the pressure is applied upward. A maximum of 50 mmHg pressure may be applied each minute for a daily 2–4 h treatment period. Too great a pressure only closes the pathways through which the fluid can escape. After learning to use the device the patient pumps his own leg at home once or twice a day. When edema persists after the ulcer heals and is not well controlled by hosiery, the indefinite use of pumping should be considered.

It must be stressed that pneumatic pumping is only a part of a total program in the control of edema. It is never a complete treatment in itself.

Local ulcer treatment

Traditional ideas about wound healing held that the ulcer should be exposed to the air and that ultimately a scab would form which would allow epithelialization to occur. Recent studies on wound healing show that the best environment is a moist one and that exposure to the air may hinder healing. This is the view presented here.

The ulcer goes through a series of changes during the process of healing. At first it is quite small with perhaps two or three small openings in the skin surface. During the ensuing week or so it breaks down, enlarging even with proper treatment. It seems that it must get worse before it gets better. There does not seem to be any way of preventing this continued breakdown. As the skin breaks down there is always a necrotic slough with enormous quantities of fluid exuding from it.

Later the ulcer bed grows velvety pink as the granulation tissue covers the base of the ulcer. Over this bed of granulation, epithelium creeps from the skin edges.

Cleansing and debriding

During the initial stage there is customarily necrotic tissue on the surface of the ulcer. There may be an actual eschar of necrotic tissue, skin, fat and fascia. Dead tissue needs to be debrided. Various enzyme ointments are touted for this purpose but are far less effective than careful surgical debridement. When the tissue is cautiously picked and snipped away there is little pain.

Wet-to-dry dressings have always been useful to debride a wound. Usually they are used during the period when the wound continues to ooze and may be more like wet soaks. If the dressing does dry out this is contrary to the moist environment approach.

Whirlpool treatments are equally popular but should be avoided unless they are absolutely essential to debridement. The major argument against their use is that the leg is dependent and without support. Dependency combined with the heat of the pool encourages further swelling in the leg.

Strong antiseptic solutions have always been popular in cleaning up the infected ulcer. Sodium hypochlorite (bleach), potassium permanganate and the mecurials should be avoided. Although they may help to clean up the dirty ulcer base they are very caustic to the surrounding tissues. The iodophor-cadamer is quite useful for the superficially infected and weeping ulcer. It is absorbent and inhibits surface infection but does not alter the healing process. If used during later stages when granulation tissue is developing, some local disinfectants actually retard the process of epithelialization.

The one topical antibiotic agent which has the least sensitizing and best antibacterial effect is silver sulfadiazine 1% (Silvadene; Hoechst Marion Roussel, Summerville, NJ, USA). It is bactericidal for many gram-negative and -positive bacteria and kills yeast. It is water soluble and easily cleaned from the skin.

There are other commercially available debriding and cleansing materials which are helpful during this stage. Washing with a bland soap and water is always good treatment. All soaps and other cleansing materials should be washed away to avoid sensitization of the skin.

Dressings

Absorptive dressings are a problem during the early exudative stage of the ulcer. Simple bulky gauze dressings are as useful as any. When removed they help to debride the wound. At this time there is enough drainage that the wound remains moist. Later when the wound is granulating and drier they should not be used.

A problem with simple gauze dressings is that the surrounding skin remains moist and soon macerates. Thus the problem becomes one of protecting the intact skin while allowing drainage of the ulcer. The new hydrocolloid dressings have helped to solve this problem. There are many excellent hydrocolloid dressings available for this purpose. My choice is DuoDERM CGF (ConvaTec; Squibb, Princeton, NJ, USA). Hydrocolloid dressings stick to moist skin and provide excellent protection as they absorb large quantities of fluid.

To create a dressing for an exudative ulcer a hole is cut in the sheet of hydrocolloid which exactly fits the edges of the ulcer. The sheet is fitted over the ulcer, pressing the dressing to seal the edges. In this way the ulcer can weep through the window while the surrounding skin is protected from the fluid. If the skin is moist and the dressing does not seem to adhere completely the pressure of the bandaging will seal it.

Some type of absorptive material is placed over the window. Gauze is satisfactory with the protective dressing on the outside skin. There are absorptive powders available as well but we like to make our own. We mix approximately equal parts by volume of zinc oxide powder with hydrophilic psyllium powder (similar to that used in bulk laxatives). The absorbent powder is heaped into the ulcer bed with a mound left over it. It is covered with a few dry gauzes to contain the powder. The leg is then wrapped with elastic bandages or a zip-up stocking. Plate 14 shows this type of dressing and the results obtained with its use.

The powder dressing is left in place as long as it is still absorbent, sometimes 2–3 days or longer. The powder seems to wick the fluid to the upper layers and even deposits the zinc oxide on open skin. This combination of powders does not seem to support bacterial growth. The powder and gauze are changed when necessary. The surrounding hydrocolloid dressing is left in place on the skin until it is soaked with fluid. Some of the hydrocolloid products are available as a powder and are used in a similar fashion.

Absorptive dressings are used as long as there is a major discharge of fluid. The leg is wrapped with one or two layers of elastic bandages from toe to knee. These conform better to bulky dressings than do limited stretch bandages or hosiery.

As the fluid discharge decreases an intact sheet of hydrocolloid may be used to cover the ulcer and surrounding skin. The fluid will first fill the ulcer space pushing the layer up to create a large bleb. It

sticks so tightly that it will continue to raise the dressing from the skin before it leaks out. It should be changed before this occurs to avoid maceration of the skin.

The thick yellowish fluid which collects beneath and interacts with the dressing has a foul odor and is often mistaken for pus. The patient should be assured that the fluid is not infected.

When the ulcer finally develops clean granulation tissue the hydrocolloid remains a perfect occlusive dressing. It maintains a moist healing environment and has been shown to stimulate the healing process. When removed carefully it will not damage new epithelial cells which are moving in from the edge. Although occlusive dressings were thought to encourage bacterial growth beneath them this has not been a problem. The treatment response to simple occlusive dressing and compression is seen in Plate 15.

When the ulcer is healed I like to keep it covered with a thin hydrocolloid. It provides protection to the fragile epithelium and maintains an appropriate degree of moisture. It can be left in place for at least a week and the patients can bathe over it, replacing the compression bandage or hose with ease.

Control of infection

The majority of ulcers are colonized by bacteria. Common surface bacteria are *Staphylococcus aureus* and *Pseudomonas aeruginosa*. Most phlebologists do not attempt treatment unless β-hemolytic Streptococci are discovered. There is little evidence to show that surface infection impedes the healing process. Most of the bacteria are growing in the exudate or eschar and disappear as healthy granulation tissue forms.

Our observations endorse this approach and show that local surface infections have little effect on healing of the ulcer bed. Topical antibacterial treatment may help to clear this colonization but may also sensitize the skin. Local infection invariably clears after the other measures of ulcer treatment are instituted.

Contrary to this viewpoint are those who believe that all new ulcers should be treated with a brief course of systemic antibiotics. This may be so but there is only anecdotal support for this approach. Needless to say, obvious cellulitis and abscess formation must be treated, even if empirically.

Care of surrounding skin

During the exudative stage we like to use large sheets of hydrocolloid to cover and protect the surrounding skin. Most of these dressings have a thin layer of waterproof plastic on the outer surface. This keeps water from soaking through from the outside but allows water vapor to escape from the skin surface. This also allows the patient to bathe with the dressing in place.

Whether the surrounding skin is moist-weeping or scaly-dry the hydrocolloid will help. It absorbs excess moisture and releases water vapor through the upper layer and retains water when the skin is dry.

When the surrounding skin is not covered by a hydrocolloid dressing it should be moisturized with a non-sensitizing lotion or cream. Some physicians like to use mineral oil to cleanse and soften the skin; I prefer water-based products although too much water causes maceration. The skin may already have become macerated from the ulcer's exudate.

Topical medications

Other than moisturizing creams topical agents should be avoided. As exception is made when the skin is so pruritic that the patient cannot keep from scratching. The patient may have already developed a neurodermatitis from scratching. The itching can be so intense in this condition that we have seen some patients pass a coat hanger beneath the bandages to scratch. In this condition a strong corticosteroid cream is applied sparingly but only until the itching is controlled.

Pharmacologic therapy

Studies in the UK and USA have shown that pentoxifylline (Trental; Hoechst Marion Roussel, Summerville, NJ, USA) increases the rate of healing of venous ulcers. The American study shows that the rate of healing is dose-related. As yet the drug is not FDA-approved for use in venous diseases.

As a hemorheological drug pentoxifylline has been used for many years to improve arterial blood flow. Its properties include increased RBC deformability with improved oxygen delivery to the tissues whereas other studies show a marked effect on WBCs. They report a reduction in WBC aggregation and activation. There may be a mild fibrinolytic effect as well. These findings support its usefulness in venous disease.

Prostaglandin E1, given intravenously, has demonstrated similar rheologic properties. Venous ulcers receiving treatment healed more rapidly than controls and were accompanied by a significant reduction of edema. Unfortunately there is no oral analogue at this time and all treatments require daily intravenous dosing.

Hydroxyethylrutosides are derived from the common black horse chestnut. We are familiar with the roasted chestnuts sold by street vendors. Although they taste good on a cold day there is no vasoactive value in this form. Oxerutins, however, are widely used in Europe as a "venotonic". The drug is said to restore the barrier properties of the fiber matrix between capillary endothelial calls. Its use improves the control of edema and helps to relieve the symptoms of venous insufficiency. A recent study shows a remarkable improvement in the control of edema with grade II compression hosiery by the addition of a commercial oxerutin. [11] However, they have not been shown to assist the healing of venous ulcers and because of their complex botanical structure will probably never become available in the USA.

Stanozolol, an anabolic steroid with marked fibrinolytic activity, has undergone extensive evaluation, also in Britain, for the healing and prevention of venous ulcers. Although it was felt at first to improve healing, careful double blinded studied have not shown any difference in healing when compared to the placebo group. Nevertheless there was demonstrable improvement of the liposclerotic skin in these patients. It tended to improve the associated symptoms of DVI as well.

Stanozolol is a steroid and the anabolic effects become marked after prolonged use. Masculinization, menstrual irregularities, headache and weight gain are but a few of the complaints from its use in women. It will probably never gain acceptance as other than an experimental drug.

Other agents are under investigation. Most are fibrinolytic agents or those which interfere with inflammatory responses of prostaglandin and peroxide production or are scavengers of free radicals. All require further evaluation to establish their possible roles in the treatment of chronic venous diseases.

At this time the only vasoactive agent which may be of assistance in the healing of venous ulcers is pentoxifylline.

Nursing assistance

A great help to us in the USA is the group of nurse specialists known as Enterostomal Therapists, "ETs". Originally they concentrated their efforts on the care of intestinal stomas. Now they have become experts in wound care. Most hospitals have a full time ET or one on call. Many ETs have a practice outside the hospital devoted to wound care. They are a useful resource and should be consulted for advice and assistance.

Role of surgery

Surgical treatment of superficial disease can start at any time. I usually wait until the surface bacteria of the leg are controlled so as not to infect other incisions. Incompetent saphenous trunks should be treated as well as their associated varicose veins. Whether incompetent perforating veins play a significant role in venous ulceration is still controversial. Surgery is hampered in the gaiter area because of the liposclerotic tissues.

Skin grafting has been used for many years to complete the healing process once granulation tissue has developed. Grafting may be essential for the healing of large ulcer defects where spontaneous epithelialization is impossible. Meshed spit thickness grafts may be needed for broad coverage. Smaller ulcers can often be satisfactorily treated with a series of "pinch grafts". Here tiny pinches of epithelium are removed under local anesthesia and applied to the ulcer bed.

Radical operations to eliminate Cockett's perforating veins were popular a few years ago, especially the Linton procedure, in which an incision along Linton's line was carried through the fascia and the perforators ligated. Long-term results in treating and preventing ulceration were disappointing. Then too the surgical sites often became infected or failed to heal, just like the ulcers they were designed to treat.

In the past few years endoscopic approaches have been used to interrupt incompetent perforators. This method allows a less traumatic entry into the subfascial space above the gaiter area and improves visualization of the perforating vessels. As a surgical technique endoscopy holds great promise. What remains to be proven is whether the treatment of perforating veins improves ulcer healing and prevents recurrence.

It should be emphasized that superficial reflux must first be eliminated before deeper treatment is considered.

Role of injection sclerotherapy

As a method of treating superficial varicosities sclerotherapy is added to other modalities. It is particularly useful in the lower leg where skin changes make surgery more difficult.

I always try to inject the varices around the ulcer area. I studied 12 patients using the Doppler in and around the ulcer. Varicose veins were injected with 0.5% STS for 2–3 treatments. In 10 of the 12 patients there was complete disappearance of flow beneath the ulcer as discerned by the Doppler. In the other two there was a marked decrease of flow. It is possible that these sub-ulcer veins represented perforating veins although it was not clear on evaluation. Nor could a

difference in healing or recurrence be determined. However, it makes good sense to obliterate as many sources of reflux as possible.

There have not been any complications occurring from the injections. The problem is that many of the varicosities are enclosed in the indurated tissue and are not visible. They can be found easily with the Doppler, marked and injected.

Platelet-derived healing factors

A number of wound care centers are extracting healing factors from platelets and other blood components. There is no consistent proof that the use of these factors improves venous ulcer healing. The greatest benefit appears with ischemic wounds such as those associated with diabetes.

Treatment of liposclerosis

There is no specific treatment for these changes. Further evaluation of pentoxifylline's effect on this condition is awaited. Stanozolol has shown beneficial effects on the induration and swelling. It is not available in the USA and its hormonal side-effects make it an undesirable agent for this purpose anyway.

Continued compression is known to soften some liposclerotic legs. Many of the changes are due to edema fluid. Continued manual drainage and mechanical compression are always helpful in shrinking and softening the leg. Some observe that pigmentation in the compressed leg will diminish.

Comments

These complications of CVI have always presented a challenge to the phlebologist. Our understanding of the histochemical, physiologic and hemodynamic changes associated with venous disease has increased immensely in recent years. Nevertheless we are left only with hypotheses regarding the causes of the dermatologic changes which develop with venous hypertension. Fibrin cuffs and WBCs remain the two most obvious suspects is this mystery. Further investigations may elucidate these questions and provide us with adjunctive treatments.

The usefulness of pentoxifylline and other pharmacologic agents awaits full evaluation. In the meantime, compression and surgery for associated incompetent surface veins will continue to be the mainstays of treatment.

References

1. Brouse NL, Burnand GJ (1982) The cause of venous ulceration. Lancet 2:243–245.
2. Homans J (1917) The etiology and treatment of varicose ulcer of the leg. Surg Gynecol Obstet 24:300–311
3. Piulachs P, Vidall-Barraquer E (1953) Pathogenic study of varicose veins. Angiology 4:59–100
4. Blalock A (1929) Oxygen content of blood in patients with varices. Arch Surg 19:898–905
5. Burnand KG, Whimster I, Naidoo A, Brouse NL (1982) Pericapillary fibrin in the ulcer bearing skin of the leg. Br Med J 285:1071–1072
6. Schmid-Schonbein GW, Usami S, Skalak R, Chien S (1980) The interaction of leukocytes and erythrocytes in capillary and postcapillary vessels. Microvasc Res 19:45–70
7. Coleridge Smith PD, Thomas P, Scurr JH, Dormandy JA (1988) Causes of venous ulceration: a new hypothesis. Br Med J 296:1726–1727
8. Coleridge Smith PD eds (1993) Microcirculation in Venous Disease. RG Landes, Austin
9. Veraart JCJM, Daamen E, Neumann HAM (1997) Short stretch elastic bandages: effect of time and walking. Phlebology 26:19–24
10. Negus D (1991) Leg Ulcers. A Practical Approach to Management. Butterworth-Heinemann, Oxford
11. Grossmann K (1997) Vergleich der Wirksamkeit einer combinierten Therapie mit Compressionsstrumpfen und Oxerutin (Venoruton®) versus Compressionsstrumpfe und Plazebo bei Patienten damit CVI. Phlebology 26:105–110

CHAPTER 10

Venous Thromboembolic Disease (VTE)

DVT is the most serious venous disease of the legs. DVT and its dreaded complication, pulmonary embolism, are collectively called "venous thrombo-embolic" disease. VTE is the third most common cardiovascular disease after ischemic heart disease and stroke. It is associated with more than 300 000 hospitalizations and at least 50 000 fatalities annually in the USA. [1]

Perhaps one-half of the fatalities are associated with an otherwise terminal illness, e.g. cancer. However, the other half have treatable diseases which would allow them to return to their regular activities were it not for the fatal embolism.

This chapter provides a brief overview of the pathophysiology of DVT, its sequelae, treatment principles and preventive measures.

Pathogenesis of deep vein thrombosis

The pathogenesis of DVT is a complex and multifactorial event. Many diverse factors have been associated with DVT: immobilization, obesity, advanced age, oral contraceptives, trauma, surgery, cancer, heart disease and stroke. Yet a perfectly healthy person can develop a DVT after a long car ride.

When seen from a teleological viewpoint thrombosis is a lifesaving feature of the circulatory system. On the other hand the thrombotic processes we are considering are inappropriate for the preservation of life. During the average day thrombosis is prevented by a delicate balance between an intact endothelium, maintenance of adequate blood flow and inhibition of activated clotting factors. [2]

Virchow's triad

Virchow in 1859 published a monumental work in which he classified the factors which he thought predisposed to the development of DVT. [3] The classic triad consists of:

- venous stasis
- venous injury
- hypercoagulability

This classification is still meaningful today and provides a framework for understanding the very complex problem of thrombosis.

Venous stasis

Stasis is not an accurate concept by today's hemodynamic standards. Nevertheless it suggests a coincidental condition in which there is an altered or diminished return of venous blood to the heart.

There are many reasons why blood may not be returned normally to the heart. Acute causes include altered muscular pumping by paralysis, bed rest, immobilization or casting of the leg. Chronic causes include prior venous disease, primary varicose veins, previous DVT with residual damage of deep or superficial systems which prevents complete emptying of the venous reservoir.

All of these factors increase the risk of developing DVT especially when other risk factors are added to them.

Venous injury

Direct vascular damage either by direct trauma, manipulation or thermal effect may initiate the process of DVT. However, there is considerable controversy whether endothelial damage and platelet aggregations are as important a factor in the formation of venous thrombus as they are in arterial thromboses.

The fact that most venous thrombi have been shown to develop in the valve cusps on an undamaged vein would tend to diminish the importance of vascular damage. It is suggested that "stasis" creates eddies of blood around the valve surfaces and thereby increases contact time with the coagulation elements. RBCs and WBCs, platelets and coagulation esterases in the presence of hypoxia are more likely to produce their coagulation effect.

Hypercoagulability

All of the factors relative to stasis and injury are involved in some way with increasing the coagulability of the blood. Tissue damage during surgery releases large quantities of thromboplastin. Decreased venous flow during recumbency can fail to wash away coagulation esterases or prevent appropriate mixing with their inhibitors. Prolonged euglobin lysis time (a measure of fibrinolytic activity) and decreased antithrombin III (AT III) levels have been reported following abdominal surgery as well.

Post-operative thrombi start at the time of surgery when all of these factors merge. It is estimated that 90% of all DVTs originate in the calf with a decreasing number beginning at higher levels. Of these, 75% remain localized or lyse spontaneously. The remainder propagate and extend proximally. These are the origin of pulmonary emboli. [2]

Hereditary hypercoagulability

It is now appreciated that many spontaneous DVTs not associated with other risk factors are due to deficiencies of normal anti-clotting factors. Among those anti-thrombotic factors are AT III, heparin co-factor II, protein C, and protein S. The most recent interest has been in factor V Leiden. This factor renders factor Va relatively resistant to degradation by activated protein C and is the most common inherited coagulation defect currently recognized. [4]

One must suspect a hereditary problem when DVT develops in a younger person with no other obvious risk factors. The possibility is greater if the patient has had a previous episode of spontaneous thrombosis and relates a family history of thromboses. Unfortunately there is usually a problem of testing for these deficiencies. The patient has already been placed on an anticoagulant which may obscure the actual deficiency. Most patients with one or more of these clotting problems are placed on life-long anticoagulants to prevent further thromboses.

Lupus anticoagulant

Lupus and other autoimmune diseases may show the presence of a circulating inhibitor of coagulation. Paradoxically these patients commonly show a clinical tendency for arterial and venous thrombosis rather than for bleeding. Some postulate that the inhibitor creates a selective interference with prostacyclin formation by the endothelium which upsets the prostacyclin/thromboxane balance. [2] It is not unusual that immune diseases such as ulcerative colitis or Crohn's disease should exhibit episodes of thrombosis in both deep and superficial systems.

Acquired hypercoagulable states

Numerous myeloproliferative states, polycythemia vera, essential thrombocytopenia, myelofibrosis and metaplasia can predispose to venous thrombosis. Diagnosis of the primary disease usually precedes the development of thrombosis. Many of these patients exhibit bleeding problems as well.

The role of exogenous estrogens in the development of blood clots has received considerable attention. Suffice it to say that thrombotic activity is dose-related. The latest birth control pills are relatively low in estrogen and may have little effect on thrombosis. Replacement doses have no effect. The effect of progestins is not clear at this time.

Pregnancy meets most of the criteria for a hypercoagulable state. However, there does not appear to be an increase of thrombotic complications during pregnancy. By contrast the post-partum period is notorious for the development of thromboembolic problems. Once called "milk leg" because the DVT appeared when the "milk came in" or "white leg" which described its appearance, post-partum DVT is now almost non-existent in the USA. Fewer babies, better prenatal care, easier deliveries, early ambulation and early discharge from the hospital have all been responsible for this change. None the less, patients who undergo Caesarean section have a higher incidence of thrombotic complications than those who have vaginal deliveries.

Many factors associated with malignancies increase

the risk of deep and superficial thrombosis. Theodor Billroth, the famous German surgeon, recognized the association of cancer and DVT. In the mid 19th century Trousseau, who himself died of stomach cancer, described the syndrome of migratory phlebitis, *thrombophlebitis migrans*, and latent malignancy. This is especially true for epithelial cancers wherein multiple coagulation factors are produced and may be released from the tumor tissue. Chemotherapy itself has been shown to increase the risk of thromboembolism.

Disseminated intravascular coagulopathy (DIC) is considered a state of hypercoagulability. Bleeding is the usual clinical result of acute DIC wherein the various clotting factors have been consumed by the widespread coagulation. In the chronic state thrombosis of large vessels may also be seen.

Development of the thrombus

As we have indicated, the nidus of the thrombus is thought to be within the cul de sac of the valve sinus where eddy currents form when blood flow is diminished. When compared to arterial thrombi the venous thrombus appears redder in color because of the predominance of RBCs and WBCs within the fibrin network. Successive layers of fibrin accumulate, into which platelets are intertwined with the RBCs and WBCs. The early thrombus is loosely attached to the vein wall by a fibrinous strand. As it collects thrombotic material it elongates and floats up into the vein lumen. If this early thrombus is not lysed it continues to propagate. As it enlarges the thrombus extends in both directions, filling the vein lumen and possibly obstructing blood flow. [5]

Thrombophlebitis

Traditionally phlebitis, an acute inflammation of the vein, was thought to initiate the thrombotic process. We know this is not necessarily true. Many thromboses can be visualized by ultrasonography where there is no inflammation present. Silent pulmonary emboli are frequent. It may actually be the growing thrombus which initiates the phlebitis. Phlebitis may be the body's inflammatory response to the thrombosis, representing an attempt to dissolve the blood clot. The term is most useful to describe the painful, red thrombosis of the superficial system.

Another term, "phlebothrombosis", has been used in the past to suggest a bland process of thrombosis with little inflammation. This term has been largely discarded.

Fate of the thrombus

It is well known that many small thrombi in the superficial veins are lysed completely with little residual damage to the vein wall or valve. This may be true in a few deep veins where the process is localized and well treated.

When there is progression the clot extends distally to the next valve or tributary or upward in a similar fashion. In some cases the "tail" can be seen waving in the flow of blood like seaweed at the water's edge. The tail or all of the blood clot may dislodge and become an embolus which can travel through the heart to the lungs. Although a dramatic result of DVT, it is probably the least common result.

Healing of the thrombophlebitic process without embolization occurs by one or more processes; lysis, canalization or organization. All are dependent on systemic thrombolytic substances as well as local factors which convert the thrombus to fibrous tissue. Although there may be temporary obstruction of blood flow during this reparative process there is seldom complete or permanent fibrous obliteration of the vein.

Clinical experience

Classically the signs and symptoms of DVT in the leg are:

- pain
- swelling
- tenderness
- erythema

Although these are the clinical signs and symptoms of inflammation and often accompany extensive DVT they are unreliable for establishing the diagnosis. For example, they are present in only half of the cases of confirmed DVT but may be present in many inflammatory medical conditions of the leg other than DVT.

Homans' sign, irritation of calf muscles with dorsiflexion of the foot, is useless in diagnosing DVT. Homans himself disowned the test but it is still used today. [6] Stand in any maternity ward and watch the nurses push the foot up as they go by the patients. By stretching the Achilles tendon this maneuver will cause pain with any inflammatory or traumatic process in the calf.

A superficial phlebitis in the absence of other venous disease or an unexplained thrombophlebitis in a pre-existing varix may be a tip-off of an underlying and silent DVT.

While not diagnostic any of these changes should initiate appropriate non-invasive testing for DVT. However, treatment for DVT should not be instituted until an objective diagnosis is made. Should a diagnosis of DVT not be made further clinical observations and examinations must be continued to explain the patient's complaints.

Establishing a diagnosis of DVT

The diagnosis of DVT must be accurate. A falsely negative diagnosis will set the patient at risk to the potential complications of pulmonary embolism and late post-phlebitic changes. On the other hand a falsely positive diagnosis of DVT will expose the patient unnecessarily to the risks of hospitalization and anticoagulation. [5]

Intravenous venography/phlebography

The venogram was at one time the gold standard for the diagnosis of DVT, but it is now being supplanted by duplex scanning in the USA. It is still widely performed in Europe and the UK.

A venogram is considered accurate only when the entire venous system is visualized. Unfortunately the dye which is injected at the foot is so diluted by blood that the iliofemoral system is often obscure. For a positive diagnosis a constant intraluminal filling defect must be seen on at least two X-ray views. If the patient has had a previous DVT his venous system may be altered by scar or stricture so as to make the venogram's evaluation difficult. [2]

Duplex ultrasonography

Duplex scanning is usually the first test to be performed for the diagnosis of DVT. Because the testing is non-invasive and painless it can be repeated as often as necessary to evaluate the progress of the DVT. If necessary it can be performed at the patient's bedside.

Ultrasonography is particularly good at visualizing the proximal large veins from the knee upward. It is these veins which are the source of most emboli to the lungs and which may not always be well visualized with venography.

Visualization of the calf veins is not always so rewarding. The expert sonographer can see most of the three large axial branches. Unfortunately many calf thromboses develop in the soleal veins which may not always be well visualized.

Like venography, ultrasonography looks at the anatomy of the veins. Initially the ultrasonographer notes that the affected vein is "too visible". It is larger than normal and stands apart from normal veins. Clots are seen as echogenic masses within the vein.

An important criterion for diagnosing DVT is the incompressibility of the clot-filled vein. A normal vein is easily compressed by the scanning head placed over the visualized vein; the clotted vein does not compress.

When results are equivocal serial testing should be considered. This may be an indication for venography especially if there is a suggestion of pulmonary embolization.

Continuous wave Doppler

The use of the Doppler is helpful during the initial assessment of the patient with a suspected DVT. It can insonate the common femoral vein at the groin, the superficial femoral vein in mid thigh, the popliteal vein at the knee and posterior tibial vein at the ankle. Because the signals may be attenuated in the normal state they must be compared with the flow patterns on the normal side. A high occlusive DVT will stop all spontaneous and phasic flow in these veins. Augmentation fails to increase flow. An isolated loss of flow in the posterior tibial vein may signal a calf vein DVT. A definitive diagnosis awaits further ultrasonographic evaluation however.

Impedance plethysmography (IPG)

IPG has been used by many as the initial screening test for proximal DVT. When positive this test demonstrates outflow obstruction of the iliofemoral system. In the past many clinicians initiated anticoagulation on its merits. Today most clinicians rely on ultrasonography for confirmation of the diagnosis or omit the IPG completely.

IPG may be useful on a serial basis to evaluate the resolution of the obstruction and to screen for recurrent DVT. [7]

[^{125}I] Fibrinogen leg scanning

This test is not widely available and requires a number of hours for completion. It has been used with the

IPG to evaluate patients with equivocal results, particularly those with suspected calf DVT. Its use is probably limited to special interest laboratories. [2]

Pulmonary embolism (PE)

A pulmonary embolus is a part or all of a thrombus which has broken away from a peripheral vein and traveled through the right heart to lodge in the pulmonary arterial vasculature. Like the DVTs from which they derive, small PEs are difficult to diagnose and large PEs obvious. PE may have few if any clinical signs or it may be so massive as to cause cardiovascular collapse with *cor pulmonale*.

Diagnosis based on clinical observation and examination is similar to that of DVT. A clinical evaluation with a presumptive diagnosis of PE is corroborated in about half of all cases.

Clinical suspicion

In my view any hospitalized patient with known DVT or positive risk factors for DVT who has any significant change of cardiac or pulmonary function has a PE until proven otherwise. Perhaps this viewpoint is extreme but PE and its sequelae may be so subtle that it goes unrecognized and untreated. In many cases the PE is the first sign of the DVT.

The classic triad of symptoms, *dyspnea, pleuritic pain* and *hemoptysis* are not always present. In the typical less-than-massive PE the patient suddenly complains of shortness of breath. Even in the absence of pain the breathing is shallow and rapid. Tachycardia may accompany the tachypnea but pain and bleeding when present develop some hours to days later. On the other hand tachypnea and tachycardia are symptoms common to many other conditions and should not be considered pathognomonic of PE.

When the embolus is massive the presenting signs and symptoms may be rather dramatic. The patient suddenly complains of severe shortness of breath accompanied with substernal chest pain. His face may become florid and he may faint. Physical findings show acute right heart failure, hypotension and altered cardiac sounds. Some patients may proceed into cardiac arrest if the outflow obstruction is significant. Prolonged hypotension may also become morbid.

Atypical presentations include unexplained fever, cardiac arrhythmias, confusion, wheezing, unexplained right and left cardiac failure and pseudo angina.

Establishing a diagnosis of PE

The situation is similar to that of suspected DVT. A positive diagnosis demands treatment with anticoagulants. If the patient has a diagnosis of DVT he is already anticoagulated and this decision is unnecessary, but if the patient does not have a diagnosis of DVT both the lungs and the legs need to be evaluated, for PE and DVT respectively. Because clinical findings and examinations are confusing and non-diagnostic, further specific studies should be instituted.

In many hospitals the initial testing is a bedside chest X-ray accompanied with pulmonary function tests and blood gases. Although these tests are easy to order and perform they are of little specific help in establishing a diagnosis of PE. Chest X-rays are often normal in the early stages of PE or at best confusing.

Radionuclide studies, perfusion scanning

Perfusion lung scanning is usually the initial testing used in most hospitals to exclude or confirm a clinical diagnosis of PE. It is a simple and safe technique of perfusion imaging which tests for pulmonary vascular occlusion. PE is virtually excluded when the test is normal, although factors can cause abnormal perfusion testing. [5]

Commonly macro-aggregates or microspheres of human albumin, in the range of 30 μm diameter, tagged with technetium-99m, are injected into a peripheral vein. Their distribution in the pulmonary arterioles is relative to the regional and local blood flow. When vascular occlusion is present from an embolus the area is not perfused with the radioactive particles. These areas appear as "cold spots" on the lung scan image.

Ventilation lung scanning

Because perfusion testing is sensitive to conditions other than PE, ventilation testing was introduced to increase the specificity for the diagnosis of PE. To perform the test the patient inhales a radioactive gas such as xenon-133. The gaseous isotope diffuses through the lower respiratory tract and gives an estimation of alveolar ventilation. [8]

Chest X-ray

Many changes have been described with PE but few are diagnostic. The X-ray is important to assess pneumonic changes and to look for other possible causes of the patient's signs and symptoms.

Selective pulmonary angiography

When other diagnostic testing fails to provide a definitive diagnosis angiography may be indicated. Using the Seldinger technique a catheter is introduced into the right femoral vein and selectively placed in each main pulmonary artery and contrast material injected. A diagnosis of PE is made when an intraluminal filling defect is seen in two or more views or an abrupt cutoff is seen in a vessel 5 mm or larger in diameter. [3]

Interpretation of testing, treatment decisions

Interpreting the results of testing is often confusing. As a result of ventilation–perfusion lung scanning the patients may be divided into two broad categories, "high probability" and "non-high probability" for PE.

If the perfusion–ventilation lung scan is in the range of high probability the diagnosis of PE is established and anticoagulant therapy instituted. However, patients who show a high probability lung scan result but a low clinical probability should undergo further investigation. This would certainly include a pulmonary angiogram if the suspicion of PE is strong in the clinician's mind. [8]

Treatment of venous thromboembolism

Objectives of treatment

- to prevent fatal pulmonary embolism
- to decrease the immediate complications of the thromboembolic event
- to prevent the recurrence of thromboembolism
- to prevent CVI from developing

Methods of treatment

- anticoagulant drugs
- thrombolytic agents
- mechanical interruption of inferior vena cava
- surgical thrombectomy in leg or lung

Anticoagulant drugs

The mainstay of contemporary treatment is anticoagulation using intravenous heparin for 7–10 days followed by 3 months of prophylactic oral anticoagulants. Heparin has an immediate effect whereas the oral agents require 3–4 days to take effect. Anticoagulants prevent the growth and extension of thrombi by inhibiting further blood clotting on the original thrombus. These agents have no significant thrombolytic activities. The body's natural fibrinolytic system is very effective in dissolving clots especially pulmonary emboli. Heparin is started intravenously after a complete blood count, platelet count, activated partial thromboplastin time (APTT) and prothrombin time (PT) are obtained.

Heparin

There are different protocols for anticoagulant intervention but a typical approach is as follows:

- heparin bolus, 5000 units intravenously
- continuous intravenous infusion, approximately 30 000 units per day

Subsequent dosage is adjusted according to the results of the APTT. The initial testing is a few hours after the beginning of treatment. The ideal level of anticoagulation is $1^1/_2$ to 2 times the APTT control.

Oral anticoagulants

Traditionally oral agents are started 5–7 days after the start of heparin treatment. However, many phlebologists prefer to start the oral anticoagulants simultaneously with the heparin, remembering that there is a 4–5 day lag period for the oral drugs to take effect. A 3–4 day overlap of the two medications is essential for continued effective anticoagulation. During this overlap period both PT and APTT are performed daily. The heparin dose is adjusted according to the APTT results and the oral anticoagulant adjusted according to the PT.

The recommended method of initiating oral anticoagulation with the coumadins is to start with the anticipated daily dosage, e.g. 5–10 mg. This is continued daily until a distinct change and direction of PT is noted. The dosage should not "chase" the day's pro-time. It is better to continue heparin longer than to stop it without having stabilized the PT for the oral drug. [5]

The goal of oral anticoagulation is to maintain the PT between $1^1/_4$ to $1^1/_2$ times normal PT, about 16–20 s when the control is typically 12–13 s.

Anticoagulant side-effects

The side-effects commonly reported for heparin treatment are hemorrhage, heparin-associated thrombocytopenia (HAT), late osteoporosis and hypersensitivity. Fortunately complications are infrequent with heparin because it is used for a relatively short time period and its effect is monitored frequently. Nevertheless one should be cognizant of those few patients who may develop a problem.

Bleeding is also the major complication of the coumadins. It is usually a result of uncontrolled dosing of the drug. The anticoagulant effect usually stabilizes after a few weeks so that the frequency of PT testing is decreased by the physician or stopped by the patient. During this time the PT may gradually increase without notice until bleeding occurs.

Vitamin K1 is used to reverse the anticoagulant effects of the coumadins. Administration of appropriate blood products, plasma or packed RBCs, will also correct the coagulation defect should there be an indication.

Dermatologic complications are also reported after prolonged dosage ranging from a mild rash to full-thickness skin necrosis.

Duration of anticoagulant treatment

Anticoagulation does not dissolve the blood clots, it only inhibits new thrombus formation. Therefore anticoagulation is continued during the period of hypercoagulability.

In the case of a first thromboembolic episode oral anticoagulation is continued for 3 months. Some physicians continue oral anticoagulation for 6 months, "to play it safe". This practice is probably not justified from the standpoint of prophylaxis and unnecessarily subjects the patient to the potential hazards of anticoagulation. Should there be extenuating circumstances which prolong hypercoagulability, such as continued bed rest or immobilization, the standard treatment program must be re-evaluated and adjusted to the individual needs of the patient.

Many clinicians treat a second episode as they would a first, i.e. 3 months oral anticoagulation. However, there is a change in attitude arising from a study which showed a 20% recurrence during the year following a second thrombus when treated for only 3 months. Therefore many second offenders are treated for a year with oral anticoagulants.

Should there be a third thromboembolic episode or evidence of a permanent congenital clotting deficiency, the treatment program should be indefinite. Patients receiving long-term oral anticoagulants should be monitored with PT every 6 weeks to 3 months after the PT has stabilized.

When DVT occurs as an isolated event in the calf muscles the risk of embolism is minimal and the customary anticoagulation program can then be altered. Compression hosiery accompanied by an anticoagulant regimen of intravenous heparin for 10 days followed by oral anticoagulants or low dose subcutaneous heparin for 6 weeks seems sufficient.

In selected cases of calf vein thrombosis no anticoagulation may be given. By necessity the calf must be re-examined frequently with ultrasonography to determine the state of the thrombus. Should it be seen to enlarge or extend, anticoagulants should be instituted.

Although the issues relating the use of anticoagulants have been addressed in a rather dogmatic manner there remain areas of controversy which have yet to be resolved. There are questions about the route and duration of heparin administration, when the oral agents should be started, and, as suggested above, the duration of oral anticoagulation. Nevertheless anticoagulation has dramatically altered the natural course of venous thromboembolism.

Thrombolytic treatment

Intravenous thrombolysis is a method of dissolving blood clots. The two thrombolytic agents that are FDA-approved for venous thromboembolism are streptokinase and urokinase. The more common of the two, streptokinase, is derived from B-hemolytic streptococci. Urokinase, as the word suggests, was first found in urine and unlike streptokinase is non-antigenic.

Three other agents, acylated plasminogen-streptokinase activator complex (APSAC), tissue plasminogen activator (tPA) and prourokinase are used for other thrombotic problems as well. Streptokinase and tPA are approved for patients with acute myocardial infarction.

Thrombolytic therapy is administered in patients with documented massive pulmonary embolism when there are electrocardiogram changes, right heart failure, persistent hypotension or deoxygenation. The objective is to prevent death by relieving the acute pulmonary outflow tract obstruction. [9]

Thrombolytic treatment should be considered in younger patients with iliofemoral obstruction less than 3 days old and when massive thrombosis causes arterial constriction and impending venous gangrene. Some clinicians believe that thrombolytic treatment should be given during all first episodes of DVT. In this way there will be lysis of thrombi before the inflammatory process has a chance to destroy or damage the vein wall and valves. The hope is to decrease permanent outflow obstruction and to preserve valvular function, two factors implicated in the development of the post-phlebitic syndrome. Some studies indicate that the late sequelae of the post-phlebitic leg, chronic deep venous insufficiency with its attendant problems, can be prevented by thrombolytic therapy. However, thrombolytic therapy is not applicable in most cases of DVT associated with recent surgery or trauma.

Interruption of inferior vena cava (IVC)

It has been obvious to many physicians that mechanically interrupting the IVC or iliac veins could completely prevent embolization from a lower thrombus. The problem has always been whether this can be done without seriously altering venous return.

External banding

During the 1960s and early 1970s there was an intense interest in vena caval interruption for the prevention of embolization of thrombi from the legs. Initially the IVC was ligated surgically, completely or incompletely occluding it. Although this approach may have prevented the transmission of emboli the procedure increased outflow obstruction, usually aggravating the original thrombotic problem. A variety of clips were then devised which tried to avoid complete occlusion. They too were surgically applied over and around the IVC to create a series of small windows through which blood but not clots could travel. The clips were often inserted at the time of surgery to prevent post-operative PE or after a series of PEs had occurred. [2]

Their effectiveness in preventing fatal embolization or decreasing permanent pulmonary damage is difficult to evaluate. Unfortunately they required a major operation, further increasing the risk. In many cases there was complete thrombosis of the lower IVC. As a result of IVC clipping, many patients later developed severe CVI in both legs. Some of the worst venous claudication, ulcerations, lymphedema and elephantiasis I have seen developed from IVC clipping. Figure 9.3 and Plate 16 demonstrate the ravages of this disease. In those cases the treatment was probably worse than the disease. With the development of intracaval filters the use of caval interruption has been abandoned.

Intracaval filters

Because of these problems with external clipping, intraluminal caval filters were developed and have assumed a prominent role in PE prevention. Two types of filters are currently in use. The Mobin–Uddin device is a fenestrated umbrella-shaped sieve. It is inserted under local anesthesia through the jugular vein. The Kimray–Greenfield device is a conical filter consisting of a series of wires which spring open after insertion. The latter is more widely used because it maintains a higher patency rate, is more versatile in its insertion site, and remains in better position. It is inserted through the internal jugular or common femoral vein in a collapsed position and opened at the appropriate position usually below the renal veins. Small hooks protruding from the base of the cone penetrate the wall of the IVC and secure it in place.

Surgical thrombectomy

In the 1950s thrombectomy became popular for acute iliofemoral thrombosis. The clot removal was assisted by the development of the Fogarty catheter, an inflatable catheter which can occlude the vein or can be used to withdraw blood clots. The high rate of fatal PE and rethrombosis caused phlebologists to look for other methods of treatment.

Nevertheless there has been a recent interest in reviving the techniques of thrombectomy for treating selected cases of acute proximal DVT. Patients who have total occlusion of the veins with clots, *phlegmasia cerulea dolens* or venous gangrene, can only profit by thrombectomy.

Recent surgical results with thrombectomy look promising. Decreased mortality and improved patency of the iliofemoral veins are reported. The improved results are thought to derive from better selection of patients, more precise information on the extent of the thrombus, the use of a more delicate surgical technique and the occasional addition of an arteriovenous fistula.

An arteriovenous fistula is constructed by attaching a portion or tributary of the GSV to the femoral artery. Arterial blood thus flushes the larger veins, minimizing rethrombosis and maintaining patency. The fistula is closed sometime later. Comparative studies using thrombectomy, anticoagulation and thrombolysis are awaited.

Pulmonary artery embolectomy

Trendelenburg first proposed surgical removal of a life-threatening PE. [10] When embolization creates a complete outflow block of the pulmonary artery death may be imminent. Thrombolysis is usually attempted first and may dissolve enough of the blood clot to allow perfusion of the pulmonary vasculature.

If not, surgical intervention may be life-saving. This involves cardiopulmonary bypass with aspiration of the clot from the pulmonary artery.

General medical care

Bed rest

Most of these patients are already hospitalized. General measures during the period of anticoagulation include attention to cardiovascular function, care of injuries or surgical recovery and hydration. Seldom is infection a problem with the thrombotic process itself. In the past antibiotics were administered in the belief that the clots were infected. This is not indicated unless there is specific evidence of infection or an associated pneumonitis.

If the patient has been ambulatory and an acute DVT develops with significant swelling he will benefit by hospitalization. This will allow continued elevation of the leg which will help decrease the associated swelling. The time in hospital is then used to initiate anticoagulation.

At one time it was thought that quiet bed rest would prevent thrombi from breaking off and embolizing. Unfortunately quiet bed rest probably increases the risk of further thrombosis. Therefore in-bed activities should be encouraged to minimize "stasis" in the affected and normal leg.

For the acute, non-hospital associated DVT ambulatory treatment with daily low molecular weight heparin and compression has been proved to be safe and effective.

Compression

During the acute phases of the thrombotic process mild compression will help attain the above objectives of edema reduction and venous return. Bed rest increases the risk of thrombosis in the otherwise normal leg. It must therefore be treated in the same fashion as the affected leg.

Wrapping of the affected leg is the best method of compression during the acute phase of thrombosis as it allows for an individualized approach to the problem of swelling. Once the swelling is controlled the leg can be measured for compression hosiery.

Prevention of thromboembolism

We have already elucidated the various risk factors which predispose to DVT. Prevention demands that we understand these risk factors and create strategies to alter them without adding undesirable side-effects.

Decrease stasis

The improvement of venous return during periods of inactivity has become a standard objective of the nursing staff. Light compression hose have become a standard for bed patients and surgical patients. The use of pneumatic pumping has increased in popularity especially with the availability of small cuffs which fit over the foot. These can be used even when a long-leg cast is in place, a situation often leading to DVT.

Low dose heparin

At the present time low dose subcutaneous heparin is the mainstay of DVT prophylaxis. A reduction of thromboembolism up to 67% by the use of this treatment has been reported.

For prophylactic use heparin is given by the subcutaneous route. In this form it is slowly absorbed and neutralizes the activated clotting factors which are formed in the hypercoagulable state. A much lower dose is required to prevent coagulation than to treat it after it has begun.

Low dose subcutaneous heparin is usually administered in 5000 unit doses injected into the subcutaneous fat at 8 or 12 hourly intervals. In the post-operative period the 8 hourly dosing has been associated with an increased frequency of wound hematomas so that 12 hourly doses may be chosen during this period. At this dosage level there is little effect on the PTT and monitoring is seldom necessary. Bleeding, although an occasional event, is much less of a clinical problem than with therapeutic doses.

Low molecular weight heparin (LMWH)

The heparin to which we are accustomed is considered unfractionated heparin (UFH). As the heparin molecule is processed it yields fractions with varying degrees of antithrombotic and anticoagulant activity. LMWH is now FDA-approved in the USA although it has been investigated and used abroad for many years. Most of the investigations have been restricted to surgical prophylaxis. The LMWH available in the USA has about one-half the molecular weight of UFH with an antithrombotic potency that is equal to or greater than UFH.

A major clinical advantage of LMWH is that all studies report a reduced incidence of bleeding. This is possibly related to its decreased inhibition of platelet function. Another tremendous advantage is an increased bioavailability which permits a once-a-day dosing regimen. The longer duration of action and minimal alteration of blood viscosity are further attributes. One prophylactic regimen uses a subcutaneous dose 2 h pre-operatively followed by a daily injection for 7 days. [9]

Studies suggest that LMWH may be preferable to UFH for certain groups of surgical patients at increased risk for DVT. A meta-analysis of orthopedic patients showed a significantly decreased incidence of DVT and PE with the use of LMWH when compared with UFH. There was also an absolute reduction is bleeding with LMWH therapy. [5]

When the two heparins were used in general surgical patients there was a significant reduction in DVT, PE and bleeding; there was little difference between the antithrombotic effects when the two agents were compared.

Ongoing investigations are in progress to determine the efficacy of LMWH in the initial treatment of DVT. One meta-analysis of nine studies indicated that LMWH, administered subcutaneously, in fixed body weight-adjusted doses is more effective than intravenous adjusted dose unfractionated heparin. If these results continue they may markedly alter the initial treatment of DVT and PE. [9]

Oral anticoagulants

Although oral anticoagulants have been shown to significantly reduce the frequency of venous thromboembolism and fatal PE after surgery, their use has not gained wide acceptance. There are a number of reasons for this hesitancy. There is a lag period for their anticoagulant effect to become stabilized, they must be monitored frequently and many post-operative patients cannot take oral medication.

Probably the major reason why oral anticoagulants have not been generally accepted is that a few episodes of major bleeding have been reported, especially when the drugs were started in the pre-operative period.

Dextran

Low molecular weight dextran, Dextran 40, is an effective prophylactic agent for general and orthopedic surgical patients. Its antithrombotic activity is related to decreased platelet adhesiveness, decreased blood viscosity and altered fibrin polymerization. Unfortunately it must be given intravenously. Usually 500 ml

are infused for 4–6 h at the time of surgery and daily for 3–5 days. Bleeding is a reported side-effect and its osmotic effect causes fluid retention. For these reasons it is not a popular prophylactic agent when heparin is available.

Anti-inflammatory drugs

Aspirin has not been a particularly effective prophylactic agent against thromboembolism. It is widely used as a prophylactic measure in the arterial system because of its antiplatelet effect. However, venous thrombosis is more commonly associated with leucocyte aggregation and aspirin is less effective for this purpose. Many surgeons also complain that aspirin causes capillary oozing during surgery.

Other non-steroidal anti-inflammatory agents are widely used to treat the associated pain and secondary inflammation of the phlebitic process.

Comments

In spite of improved medical care thromboembolic disease is a continuing problem especially with patients undergoing general and orthopedic surgical procedures. Because of the enormous numbers of successfully treated surgical patients without DVT the problem seems quite distant until one remembers the 50 000 deaths each year in the USA from PE.

At times thromboembolic disease goes unnoticed or is self-limiting. Resolution may be complete with no late sequelae, but the complications are so devastating that prophylaxis should be considered for patients undergoing surgical procedures with an exaggerated risk for DVT and PE. Victims of major trauma should also be considered at high risk.

There is some recognition by the medical community of these issues, as shown by the placement of antithrombotic hose on hospital patients. Ideally each patient undergoing major surgery should be evaluated for DVT risk factors as they are now evaluated for cardiovascular risks. At surgery they would all have some type of intermittent pneumatic compression placed on their feet or legs.

The availability of LMWH with its ease of once-a-day subcutaneous administration and minimal bleeding may change our attitudes in this regard.

References

1. Anderson FA, Wheeler HB, Goldberg RJ et al (1991) A population-based perspective of the hospital incidence and

case-fatality rates of deep vein thrombosis and pulmonary embolism. Arch Intern Med 151:933–938

2. Brouse NL, Burnand KG, Lea Thomas M (1988) Diseases of the Veins. Pathology, Diagnosis and Treatment. Arnold, London

3. Virchow R (1859) Die Cellular Pathologie. August Hirschwald, Berlin

4. Ridker PM, Miletich JP, Hennekens CG, Buring JE (1997) Ethnic distribution of factor V Leiden in 4047 men and women; implications for venous thromboembolism screening. JAMA 277:1305–1307

5. Hull RD, Raskob GE, Leclerc JR (1985) The diagnosis of venous thrombosis in symptomatic patients. In Recent Advances in Blood Coagulation, Poller L ed. Churchill Livingstone, London, pp 35–61

6. Homans J (1944) Diseases of the veins. New Engl J Med 231:51–57

7. Hull RD, Secker-Walker RH, Hirsh J (1987) Diagnosis of Deep Vein Thrombosis. Hemostasis and Thrombosis, 2nd edn. Lippincott, New York, pp 1220–1239

8. Gaschman PC (1984) Pulmonary angiography. Clin Chest Med 5(3):465–477

9. Leclerc JR (1992) Practical Guide to Thromboembolic Disorders. DuPont Pharmaceuticals, Mississauga, Ontario

10. Trendelenburg F (1908) Uber die operative Behandlung der Embolie der Lungenarterie. Arch Klin Chir 86:686–692

Color Plate Section

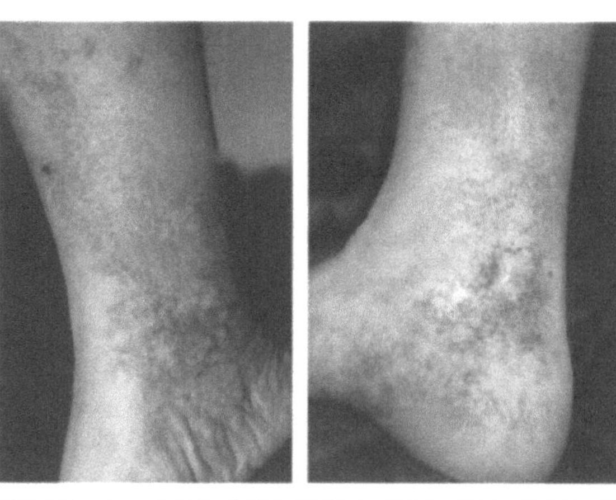

Plate 1 These two examples of white atrophy occurred in patients whose biopsies showed "fat atrophy". They were treated unsuccessfully with intralesional steroids. Phlebologic evaluation demonstrated greater saphenous vein reflux. Appropriate treatment cured the dermatologic condition.

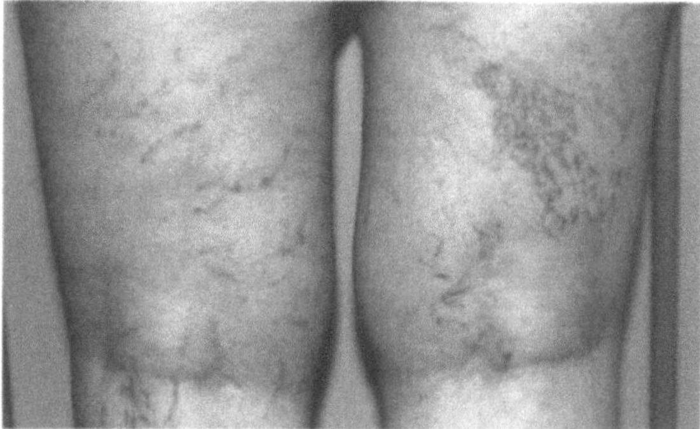

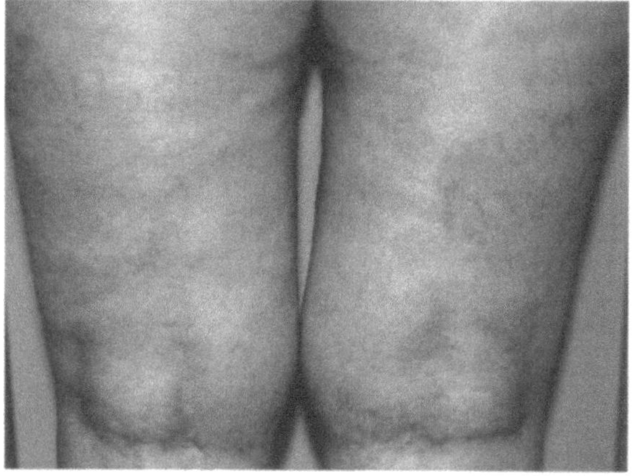

Plate 2 The upper photograph shows a typical grouping of telangiectasias which emanate from incompetent reticular veins in the thigh. Treatment required six sessions using 0.3% sodium tetradecyl sulfate. The lower photograph shows the results 6 months later. Although most of the spider veins have been eliminated some still remain. There was intense pigmentation which lasted for almost 4 months.

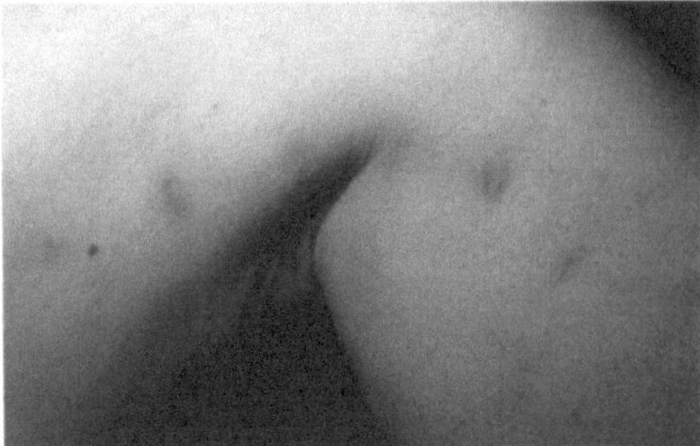 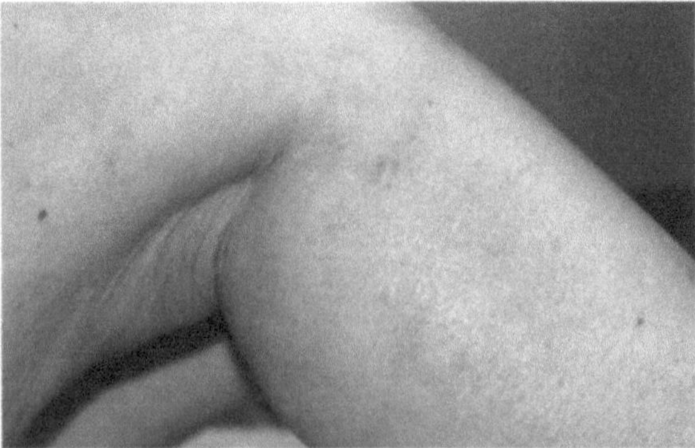

Plate 3 The photograph on the left was taken 4 months after microincisional phlebectomy of a large lateral thigh vein. The scars resulted from 4–5 mm incisions which were used in our early experience. The photograph on the right was taken 4 years later. One small scar remains below the knee.

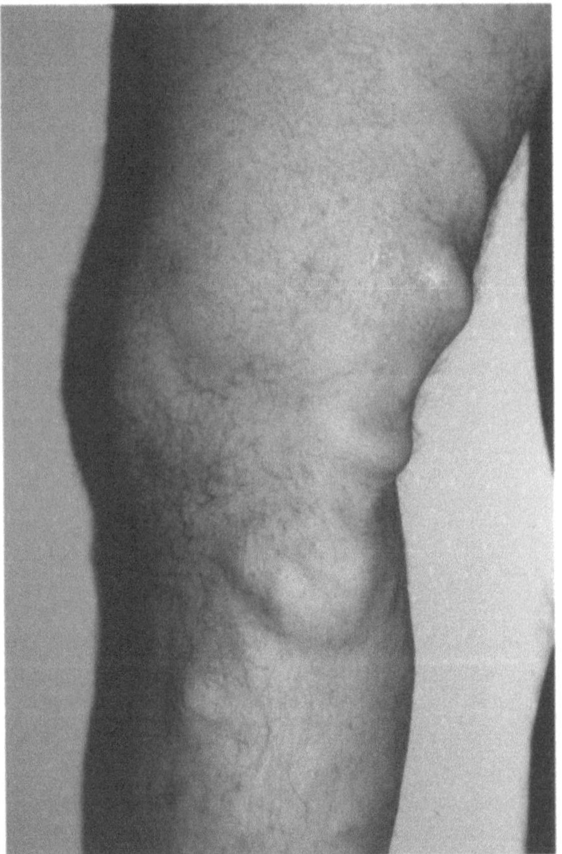 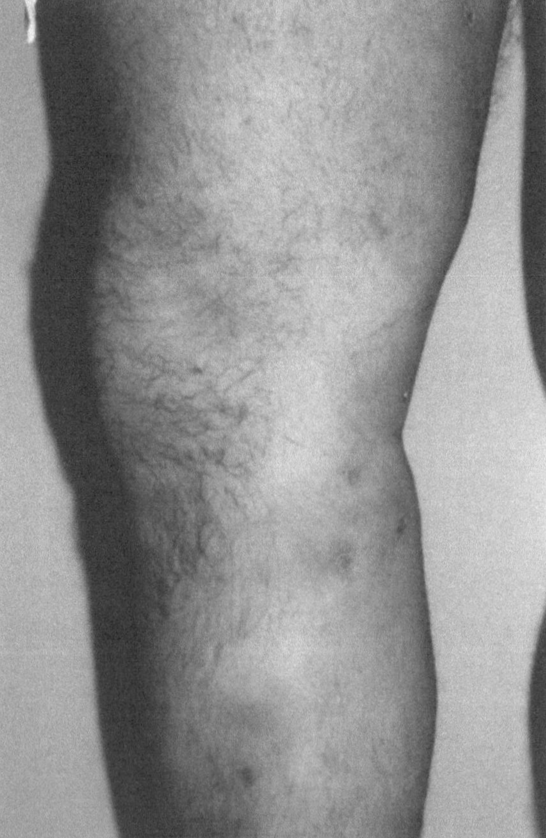

Plate 4 The greater saphenous vein was dilated to more than 3 cm in this patient. He had ulcerations on the shin and ankle as well as thickening and darkening of the skin for more than 20 years.

Plate 5 This photograph was taken 2 weeks after surgical removal of the greater saphenous vein. Because of dense fibrosis a phlebectomy technique was used to excise the vein. Small scabs can be seen overlying the 4–5 mm incisions needed to remove the vein. His ulcers healed and have remained so during the following 5 years.

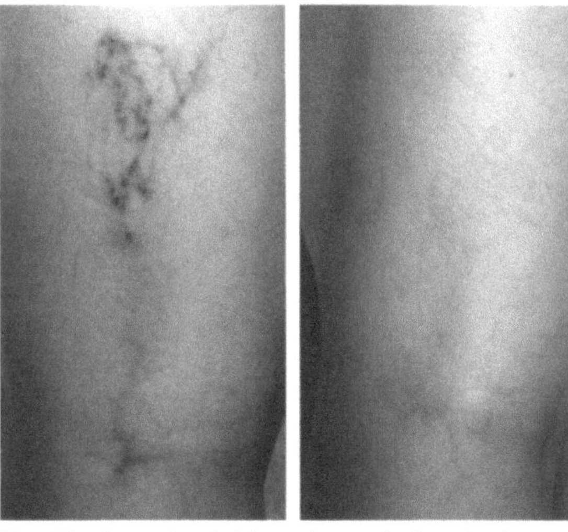

Plate 6 The photograph on the left was taken 4 weeks after an initial treatment of blue and spider veins with 0.3% sodium tetradecyl sulfate. Trapped blood was evacuated on this visit so that 2 months later (right) all pigmentation had disappeared.

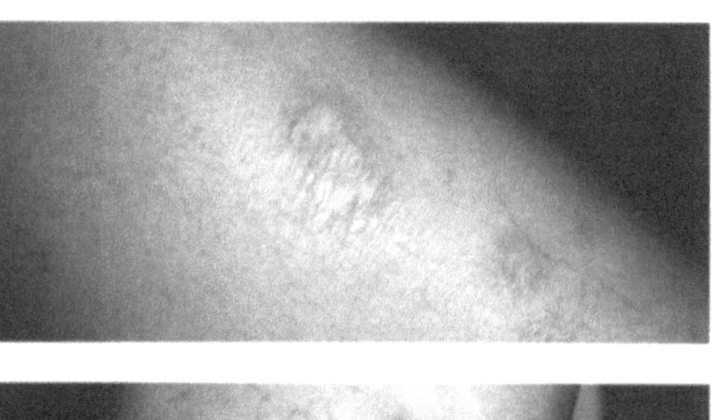

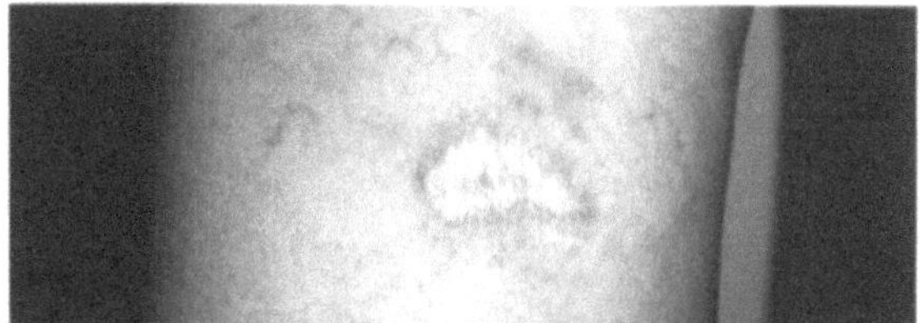

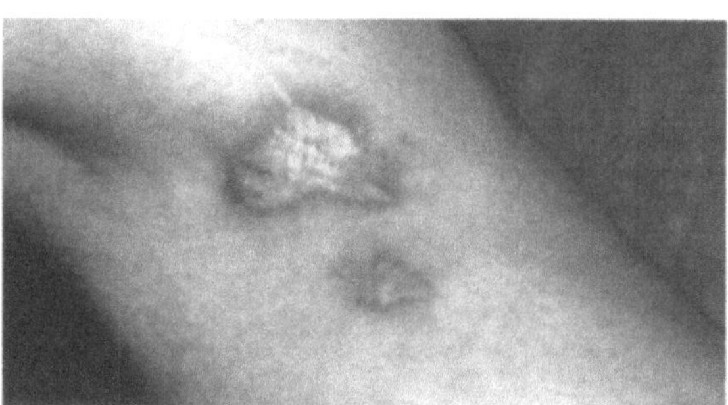

Plate 8 Three photographs show the devastating side-effects of injected sclerosants. All of the legs had been treated with hypertonic saline by other physicians. The details of treatment are unknown. Nevertheless there were deep burns to the skin with permanent scars present 3–6 years after treatment.

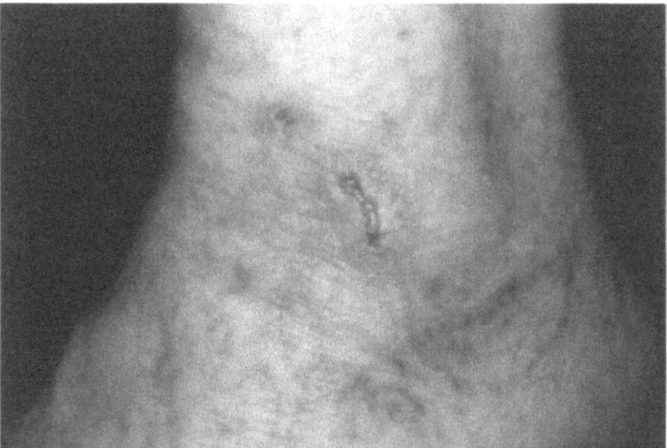

Plate 7 This patient had received three treatments of 0.3% sodium tetradecyl sulfate on both legs without incident. Following the fourth treatment this shallow ulceration developed on the ankle. It healed in 3 weeks without scarring but was quite painful during this period. Only occlusive hydocolloid dressings were used in its treatment.

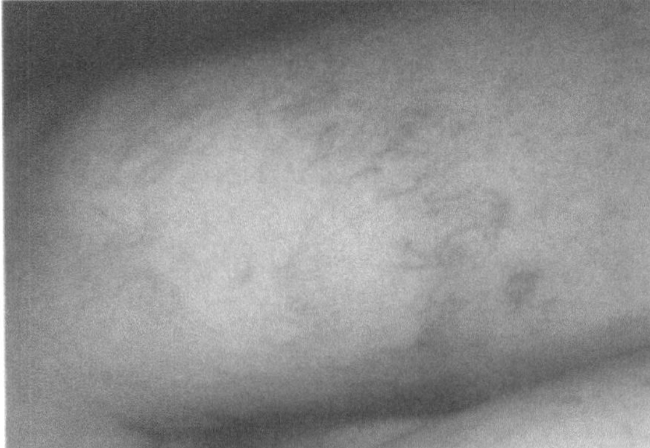

Plate 9 Repeated treatments of associated blue and spider veins usually cause no problems. Nevertheless this post-inflammatory matting developed on the inner thigh after three treatments using 0.6% polidocanol.

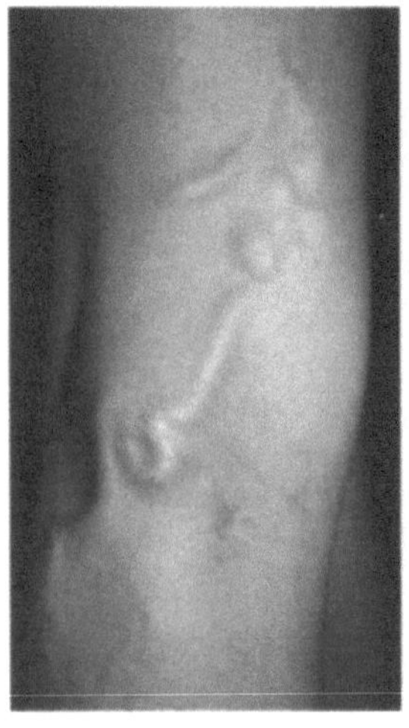
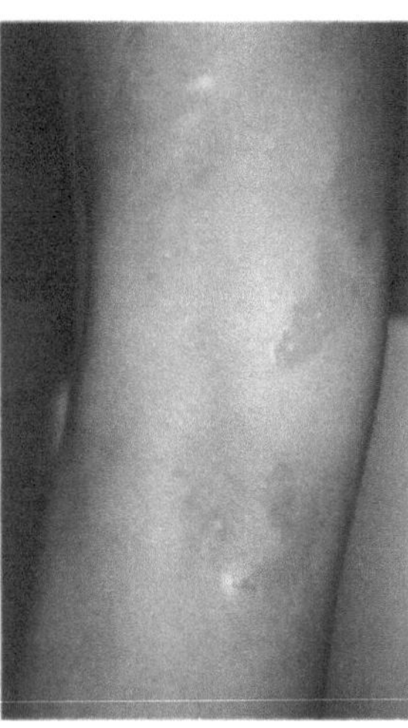

Plate 11 This complex of varicose veins in the popliteal area originated from an incompetent greater saphenous vein (GSV). The varicose vein measured 1.3 cm in diameter and was treated after reflux had been corrected in the GSV. Two sessions of injections using 0.75% sodium tetradecyl sulfate and compression were needed to sclerose it. Four months later (right) discoloration had disappeared and the vein was completely flattened.

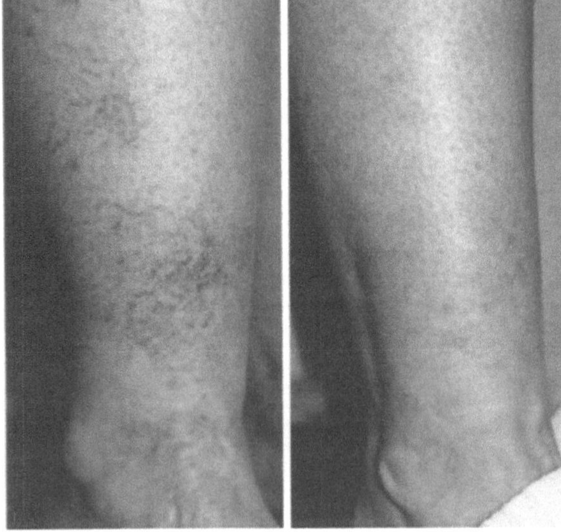

Plate 10 The example on the left represents a typical grouping of pebbly telangiectasias, "blue blebs" around the ankle. This is the same patient seen in Plate 2. Their eradication required six treatments with 0.3% sodium tetradecyl sulfate. There was intense pigmentation for 4 months. The photograph on the right was taken 6 months after treatment with some pigmentation still present.

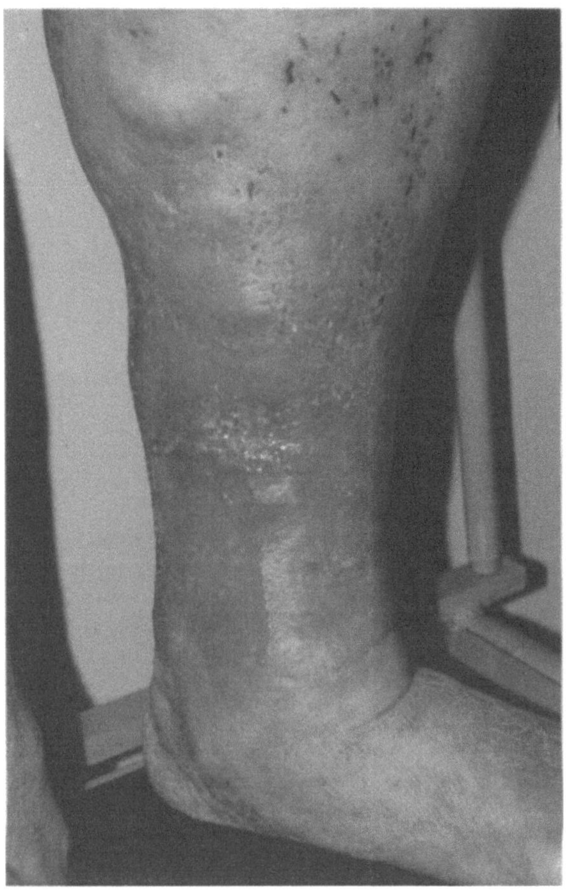

Plate 12 *(Right)* This leg, also shown in Fig. 3.2, demonstrates most of the features of chronic venous insufficiency. The patient presented with acute lipodermatosclerosis, seen here as the bright red inflammatory reaction in the skin. Healed excoriations are present from the intense itching and resultant scratching. Clear fluid is trickling from the shallow ulcer.

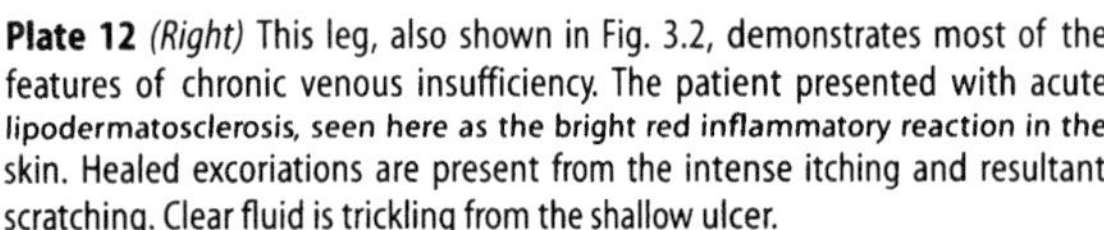

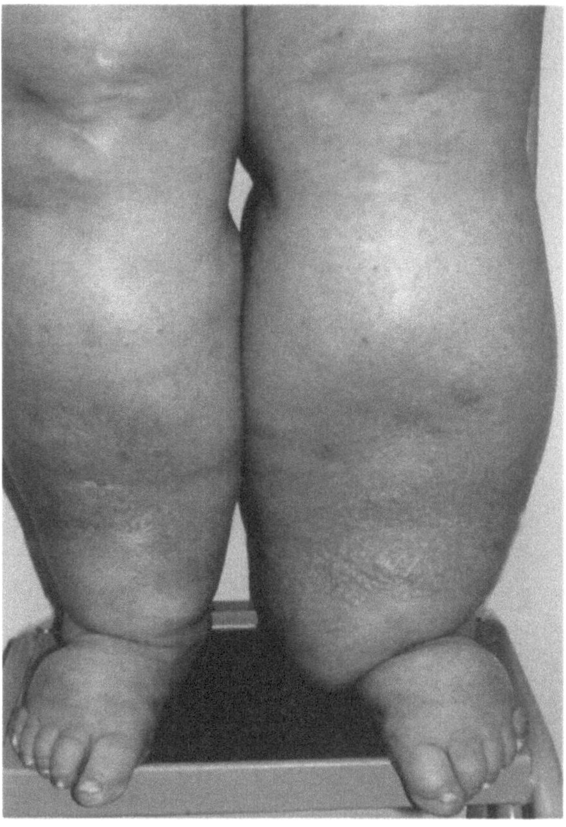

Plate 13 There is little question about the diagnosis in this case. The edematous feet and toes and hugely swollen calves can only be hereditary lymphedema. The skin is taut and does not "pit". Papillary changes are beginning in the lower calves with inflammatory skin changes above them.

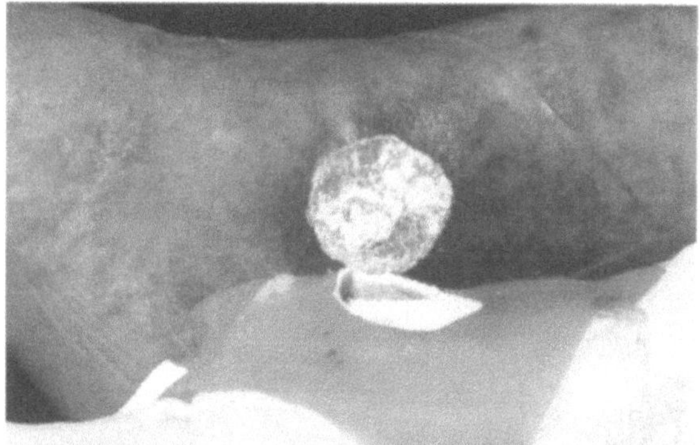

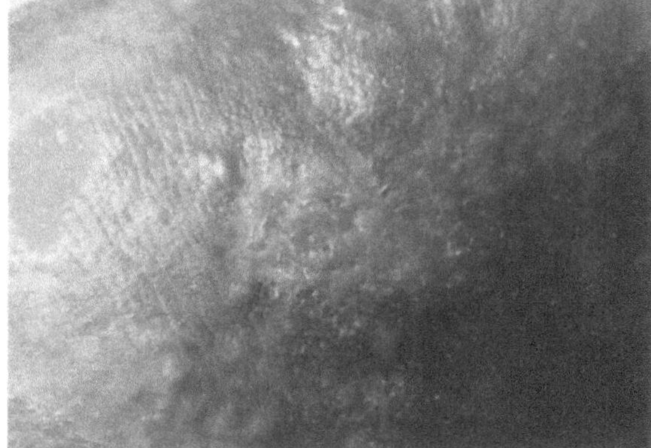

Plate 14 The upper photograph shows the type of dressing used for exudative ulcers. The hydrocolloid dressing has a hole cut in it for drainage to the absorbent powder. The surrounding skin has been protected by the dressing. The lower photograph demonstrates the effectiveness of treatment which used only a hydrocolloid dressing and compressive wrappings. Epithelium is resurfacing the granulating ulcer base, which is healed after 3 weeks.

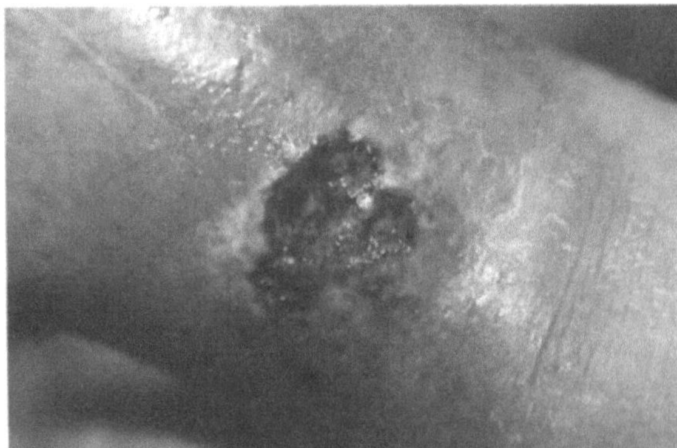

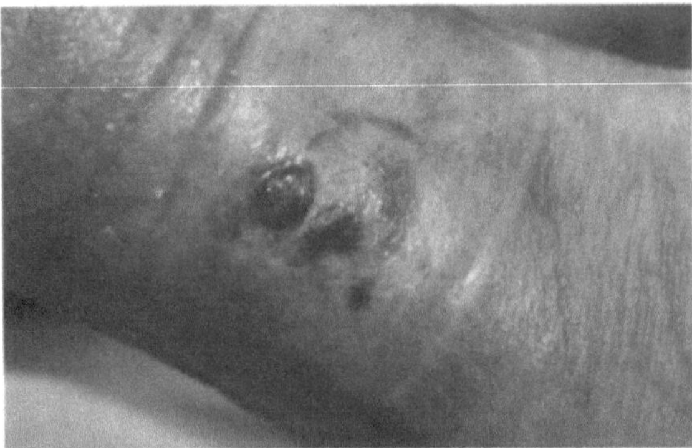

Plate 15 The upper photograph shows a fresh, untreated ulcer coming from an incompetent lesser saphenous vein. There is purulent debris in the ulcer, which is surrounded by acute inflammation. The lower photograph was taken 5 weeks after treatment with compression bandaging. There is a marked decrease of inflammation and infection and an observable healing of the ulcers.

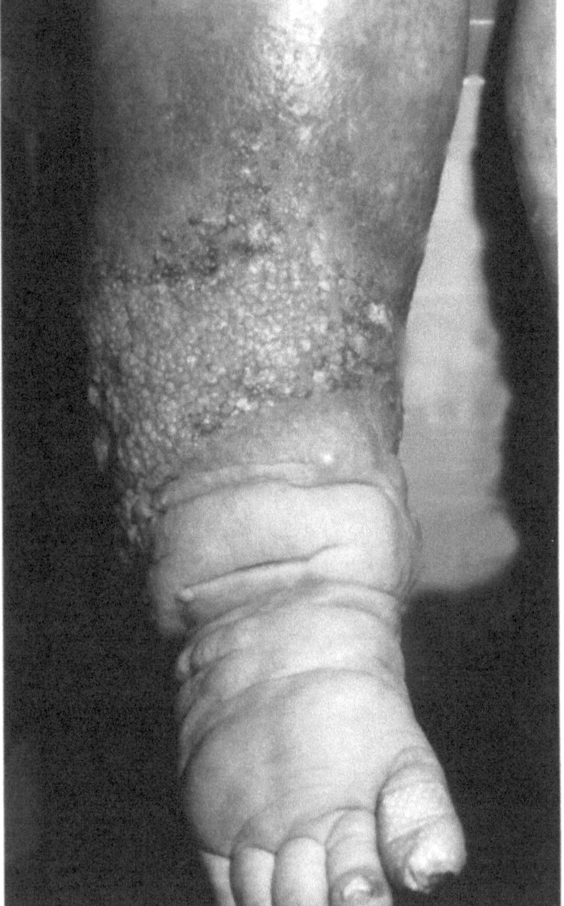

Plate 16 This unfortunate patient had a deep venous thrombosis following childbirth in 1967. The inferior vena cana was interrupted by clipping to prevent pulmonary embolization. Early edema changed to lymphedema and later elephantiasis. Papillomatosis, deep ulcerations, "intractable" swelling and pain confined the patient to her home. A year of combined treatments – manual lymph drainage, wrapping, compression bandaging and hosiery – were needed to heal the ulcers. For the first time in 20 years the patient can wear ordinary shoes and go to church.

Index

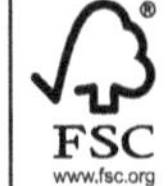